PRIMETIME BODIES

· · · · · · · · · · · · · · · ·

THE SIX-WEEK HOLLYWOOD FITNESS PROGRAM

· · · · · · · · · · · · · · · ·

CYNTHIA TIVERS AND KATHY KAEHLER

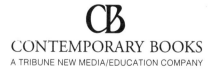

CONTEMPORARY BOOKS

A TRIBUNE NEW MEDIA/EDUCATION COMPANY

Library of Congress Cataloging-in-Publication Data

Tivers, Cynthia.
    Primetime bodies : the six-week Hollywood exercise program /
Cynthia Tivers and Kathy Kaehler.
       p.   cm.
    ISBN 0-8092-3281-2
    1. Exercise.   2. Physical fitness.   I. Kaehler, Kathy.
II. Title.
GV481.T58   1996
613.7'1—dc20   95-41471
                                            CIP

Cover design by Amy Nathan
Cover photos and interior exercise photos by Harry Langdon
Interior design by Frank Loose Design

Published by Contemporary Books, Inc.
Two Prudential Plaza, Chicago, Illinois 60601-6790
Manufactured in the United States of America
International Standard Book Number: 0-8092-3281-2

10   9   8   7   6   5   4   3   2   1

To Bella and William Kandelman . . . my loving parents, whose gifts of life and laughter give me everlasting inspiration.

And to Dani, a beautiful beam of light even on the darkest days.

Cynthia Tivers

To my junior high gym teacher, Miss Bobbie Jo Reider, for her inspiration . . . She was the coolest gym teacher anyone could have had.

To my parents, who always found time to get me involved in sports . . . especially my ever-patient mother who sat through all those two-hour dance classes.

And to Billy, my husband, thank you for your patience. I love you.

Kathy Kaehler

Contents

Acknowledgments

The authors would like to thank all the people who contributed their prime time and talent to help make this book a reality. Thanks to Stan Corwin for his enthusiastic response to the idea for this book and his unwavering support from start to finish; to Kara Leverte for her center-stage role as our extraordinary editor; and to Harry Langdon, who has cast his talented photographic eye on Hollywood's most beautiful women and who has now added us to his prestigious list.

We would also like to thank Dr. Frank Hilf, whose unwavering computer support helped these printed words appear on the page. And we want to thank all our celebrity clients who shared their motivating stories with us. Thanks to all of you.

Introduction

In 1987, Kathy Kaehler auditioned for a job with Jane Fonda. Jane was about to open her exclusive spa, Laurel Springs Retreat, and she was looking for a director.

Kathy had been setting up wellness centers in Denver when she got the call to come to Santa Barbara to meet Jane. A competitive athlete since grade school, Kathy thought the challenge of designing a fitness program for a health spa run by the already legendary fitness star was something she had to try. It was a role that had great potential.

The audition lasted a full day and included long talks and plenty of exercise. In addition to Kathy's leading Jane through a low-impact aerobics class, Jane took Kathy on her routine two-mile hike in the Santa Barbara Mountains where her ranch was situated.

It was a good opportunity for the two fitness experts to get to know each other and determine if they were a fit. Jane found that Kathy was the woman she was looking for and Kathy found the woman whose path she would follow—starting right there—straight up the mountains. Despite the twenty-five-year age difference between the two women, Jane had Kathy huffing and puffing behind her for two hours. Kathy got a superstar dose of inspiration. To this day, Kathy has never forgotten how hard it was to climb that mountain, how important it was for her to prove that she could do it, and how rewarding—from that day forward—it's been for her life.

Kathy became the program director for Laurel Springs Retreat. Through her work there she met Melanie Griffith and eventually left Santa Barbara to become Melanie's private personal trainer. Through her work with Melanie and some of Melanie's friends, Kathy started taking on other celebrity clients who admired what Kathy had done with their friends' fitness levels.

Kathy has managed to break sweat at one time or another with everyone from Barbra Streisand and Farrah Fawcett to Meg Ryan and Michelle Pfeiffer. And let's not forget Candice Bergen, Julianne Phillips, Claudia Schiffer, Penelope Ann Miller, and of course, Jane Fonda and Melanie Griffith. Then there are the men in her professional life: Sugar Ray Leonard, Tom Arnold, Andrew McCarthy, and Rob Lowe.

Not bad for a kid from Detroit who was born with a dislocated hip. Delicate surgery corrected her problem, however, and gave her a chance at a normal life.

While it's part of Kathy's job to keep her clients motivated, Kathy has found that many of her star clients inspire her. Here are a few examples.

Michelle Pfeiffer mentioned this about working out: "Even if I have only five or six hours to sleep every night and I have to choose between an extra hour of sleep or an hour to work out, I will choose to work out. It gives me far more energy and stamina throughout the day than the extra sleep would."

Kathy knows how hard Michelle works. It's not unusual for her to have twelve-hour workdays when she's shooting a picture. And when she's not filming, she's fulfilling the demanding roles of a wife and mom. Still, when Kathy shows up at her door at five in the morning, she's ready to go.

We find Michelle's attitude personally inspiring.

Meg Ryan is another example of focus and determination. About a year after Meg had her baby, Kathy and Meg started running. After running less than two miles, they'd walk. For about three months they kept increasing the mileage until it seemed as if all of a sudden Meg was running eight miles in less than an hour. That's tough work—especially after a pregnancy. Kathy had to work just as hard as Meg did. All Kathy could do was marvel at how this talented actress could be as focused on her workout as she was on her work.

And then there's Julianne Phillips. When Kathy gets to Julianne's house to work her out, Julianne has a baked potato in the oven and vegetables steaming in liquid aminos—she's got a healthy lunch all planned out for right after their workout session. Julianne's organization contributes greatly to her commitment to a healthy lifestyle.

There are many other examples that we will share with you throughout this book. But first we would like to let you in on a few other inside notes.

I worked with Kathy on the exercises used in the six-week program and burned the midnight oil organizing and researching Kathy's notes to come up with the prose you are reading.

As an exercise and fitness devotee and author of another exercise book, I also had the experience necessary to recognize Kathy's incredible talent and knowledge. I convinced her to share her expertise with you.

The basis for the six-week program (as well as the personal training stories) comes from Kathy's successful work with her celebrity clientele as well as from the years she spent teaching exercise classes. You can be sure that whatever moves you make, Michelle, Meg, Melanie, Claudia, Julianne, and others have tested the waters for you.

The program we've designed for you is basic and classic. But don't let that mislead you. The routines are challenging and effective. The workout should take you about 25 minutes to do. The warm-up takes between seven and eight minutes. All you need is a sturdy chair and a carpeted floor or exercise mat, music, and a good attitude.

Our workout will shape you, tone you, and make you feel really good about yourself. If you want to lose weight as you gain shape, follow a diet that is low in fat and high in fiber. Count your calories, too. The fundament of weight loss is to take in fewer calories than you expend. There's no magic, just good sense and dedication to your goal of looking and feeling great.

We hope that you dedicate the next six weeks to working with us as we take you through our program. We promise you results if you promise to keep your appointments with us.

If Michelle Pfeiffer can do it on five hours of sleep, think what you can do. Wouldn't it be great to look as good as she does?

Cynthia Tivers

1

Primetime Shape-Up
Scripting Your Program

Almost anything can happen in the movies. . . . Ugly ducklings turn into swans, the good guy always wins, the hero gets the girl, the women are always gorgeous, and of course, love conquers all. But have you ever noticed—no one ever sweats?

Well, they do when you're not looking.

There is great magic in the movies, and the stars we love to love are our ideals because of their extraordinary beauty and talent. But there isn't very much magic in how they get up there on the silver screen. It's hard work. Mother Nature gives birth, and baby, it's up to you to nurture Mother's gift.

No one knows that better than actors whose professional lives are as dependent on their looks as on their talent. The competition for roles is fierce, and the reasons are obvious. The payoff to success in Hollywood is legendary.

There is no question that talent is the *sine qua non*. But after that, beauty and hard work are the top requirements. And in today's Hollywood, beauty doesn't stop at the neck. It's practically a requirement for stars to have beautiful and healthy-looking bodies. In fact, working out regularly is such an important part of the success equation that top actresses will even wake up in (what most of us would consider) the middle of the night, to start their day exercising.

1

It takes a lot of dedication, fortitude, and tenacity to create a primetime body. But actors know that being in better-than-great shape often means the difference between getting the part and not getting the part. For instance, in *Indecent Proposal,* would Robert Redford's character have paid a million dollars to sleep with a woman who didn't look as great as Demi Moore? Or could you imagine anyone in less than the great shape Melanie Griffith was in believably declaring to Harrison Ford in *Working Girl*, "I have a bod for sin and a head for business"?

Having a bod for movies was definitely a primary asset for both Demi Moore and Melanie Griffith when they were cast for the roles in *Indecent Proposal* and *Working Girl*. And having a great body in Hollywood these days doesn't mean having just a thin body; it means having a toned and shapely body that's healthy and fit.

YOU'VE GOT TO TALK THE TALK . . .

Actors have language that communicates their craft and technique as they work to achieve their goal. All movie actors know the *cheat shot,* which fools the audience into believing something's happening when it's not. For example, a character jumps off of a building but is really landing on a mattress just below her and out of sight of the camera.

You can't cheat, however, when it comes to giving a great performance. It takes focus; it takes dedication; and it takes being true to the character the actor is portraying. Working out carries the same requirements.

For the actor, words such as "motivation," "objective," "visualizing," and "instrument" are all integral parts of her vocabulary. They're words that work for working out, too, and we'll be using these acting terms as we go through our six-week exercise program.

We've chosen to do this because our six-week program will teach you what it takes to make you as confident as any actor to stand in the spotlight of your own life. We all deserve to take center stage in life. No matter what our careers are, we can all have primetime bodies. Just as an actor prepares for a part in a show or movie, we have to prepare for our part as primetime bodies— that is, being in the best shape we can be in.

The actor's body is her "instrument." She uses it to express emotions, to communicate thoughts, to make statements about who she is. Like any instrument it has to be played with skill and artistry for its full potential to be realized.

Your body is your instrument, too. The shape your body is in tells stories about you long before you get the chance to say a word. The more motivated you are to get it in good shape, the better chance you'll have to confidently take center stage in your own life.

. . . AND WALK THE WALK

We believe, based on our years of experience, that in order to make a change in the way your body looks, you have to work out at least four times a week. If you want to make exercise a permanent part of your lifestyle, plan on working out four to six times a week. Limiting yourself to one or two workouts per week will slow the results, and you'll have too many other days to which you can push off your commitment. If you work out four to six times a week, it becomes a regular part of your life and you'll make quicker and more lasting changes in your body.

You'll also need to figure out when you should work out. We recommend treating your exercise like any other appointment. Write it on your calendar so you have dedicated time. Keep your appointment no matter how hard your day was or will be, no matter whether you're at home or on the road, whether you feel like it or not. If you still feel like making an excuse, stop and think about Michelle Pfeiffer.

When she was shooting *Batman*, her shooting schedule was so demanding that we worked out at 4:30 in the morning, five days a week for six months. Michelle made our workouts part of her schedule, gru-

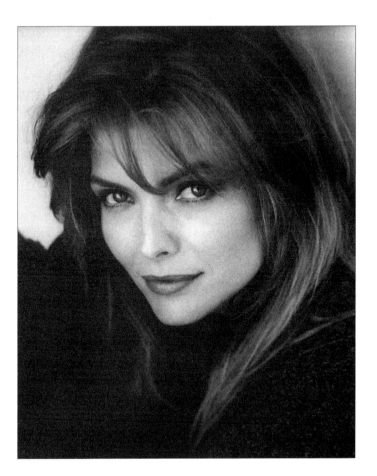

eling as it was, and she never made excuses.

When she shot *Age of Innocence* she worked in New York. We faxed her a workout every night. It would be put under her door and in the morning she'd follow that workout before she left for the set.

For her latest movie, *Up Close and Personal,* we went back to our early morning workouts. We showed up every day at her house at 5 A.M. and worked out until 6:00. At 6:15 the studio had a car waiting to take her to the location where they would shoot for the day.

It all starts with organization and motivation. Michelle has made working out part of her lifestyle. It doesn't matter if her trainer is there to push her. Michelle pushes herself. Even when she's working on a film, it's so important to her to work out that she just gets up earlier to fit it into her day. She doesn't think about how much energy it takes to work out in the morning, but rather, Michelle says that exercising gives her energy for the day.

Most of us lead busy lives. If you organize and prioritize you can be as successful as Michelle is in getting your workout done. And we've made it easy for you to start.

THE SCRIPT

We've come up with a workout program that should take you between 20 and 25 minutes to complete. We'll be using exercises that will work both your upper and lower body. All you need to begin is a chair and, if you don't have carpeting, a pad for your knees.

We have a warm-up and cooldown for you to follow. If you prefer (and we suggest you try), do at least 20 minutes of your favorite cardiovascular exercise each time you start our program. If you can't do your own, start with our warm-up routine. But remember—always warm up your muscles before you work them out. Warming up reduces the risk of injury and makes the exercises more effective.

Physiologically, exercise in the morning is more effective because when you stimulate your metabolism earlier in the day your body burns its fuel (food) more efficiently the entire day. Most people feel more energetic for the rest of the day after working out early.

But if you're the type of person who can barely brush her teeth first thing, try working out during your lunch hour. We did that with Marsha Mason and Jamie Gertz when they were working on a sitcom at Columbia. They would order their lunch in the morning and it would arrive while we did a 45-minute workout on the set. Then they'd quickly change, eat their lunch, and go back to work.

If you find that the only time you can set aside to work out is at night, then do it at night. Just don't eat a big meal afterward and then go to sleep. Try eating before you work out—a half hour to one hour before you exercise. Then, if you need to, eat a light-carbohydrate snack or a piece of fruit after your nighttime workout, before you go to sleep.

Consider your appointment book the script you're going to act out each day and make sure your action includes your workout. If you want to have a primetime body, you've got to play the part. Any actor going for a good performance makes sure her script works for her—make sure yours works for you.

2

Anatomy

Getting the Parts

It takes muscle to make it in Hollywood. That muscle may be packed on Sylvester Stallone or Arnold Schwarzenegger or it could be sculpted on Jamie Lee Curtis or Julianne Phillips.

No matter who's wearing them, well-toned bodies are shaping their parts both on-screen and off. As we take you through the next six weeks we're going to put your muscles through a program inspired by our celebrities as we train their primetime bodies.

We're going to work out skeletal muscles from your head to your toes. But before we work them out we'd like to help you "get" your parts by giving you some muscle "back-story."*

There are about 700 muscles in the human body. Men and women have the same number of muscles but men do carry more of their body weight in muscle. About 42 percent of a man's weight is muscle and about 36 percent of a woman's weight is muscle. While the number of fibers in a muscle is the same for men and women, men develop stronger and bigger muscles than women do because of the male hormone testosterone, and also because proportionately, their muscles are longer and are stretched over longer

---

*Back-story is the history behind a character which makes the character who she is at the time the story (movie, play, or TV show) takes place.

bones, which gives them a mechanical advantage.

But women can improve their muscle strength through weight training. Strength training involves performing a body motion while you add resistance to that motion. Muscles get stronger or weaker in response to demands placed on them. Muscles lose strength when they're not used and they gain strength according to the load placed on them. As the muscle gets stronger, it has to be challenged harder in order to keep developing. So during our six weeks, as your muscles adapt to a given exercise resistance, we will suggest you increase the resistance by using weights.

Why should women develop their muscles? First and most basic, less fat and more muscle gives you a leaner, firmer, and fitter appearance. Muscle burns more calories than fat. Even when we're asleep, our skeletal muscles (the ones we'll be training) are responsible for more than 25 percent of our calorie use.

In addition, bones grow denser from stress placed on them. So weight-bearing exercises, like many of the exercises we'll be doing, will help stem osteoporosis.

People who don't train their muscles through exercise lose about one-half pound of muscle every year, starting in their late 20s. That gradual loss of muscle tissue means adults who don't train will reduce their metabolic rate* by one-half percent every year. This gradual decrease in metabolism is closely related to the gradual increase in body fat that we all face as the years go by.

So body muscle not only makes you look good now, but it will also allow you to eat more and gain less weight as you go through life.

Now let's take a look at the major muscles we'll be working over the next six weeks. Starting at the top:

DELTOIDS These are your shoulder muscles. They're used mainly to raise your arm. We'll use them every time we work out. We'll be working the anterior deltoids (at the front of your shoulder), the posterior (the back of your shoulder), and the middle deltoid (at the top). The deltoids form the shoulder cap.

PECTORALS Chest muscles that help the shoulders move and are themselves used when you push on things. For women, well-developed pectoralis muscles help your breast area

---

*Metabolism is the rate at which your body burns calories for energy. The basal metabolic rate (BMR) is the amount of energy it takes to support the metabolic work of the body's cells. This includes beating of the heart, respiration, and the maintenance of body temperature. The body must first use its energy to support these basic functions before calories can be used for any other activities including exercise.

Muscles:
THE VIEW FROM
THE AUDIENCE

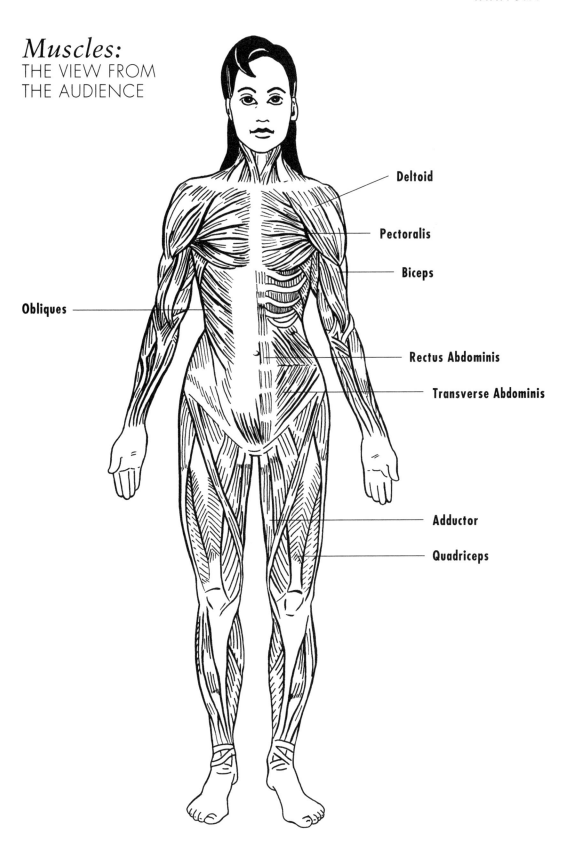

Deltoid

Pectoralis

Biceps

Obliques

Rectus Abdominis

Transverse Abdominis

Adductor

Quadriceps

Muscles:
THE VIEW FROM BACKSTAGE

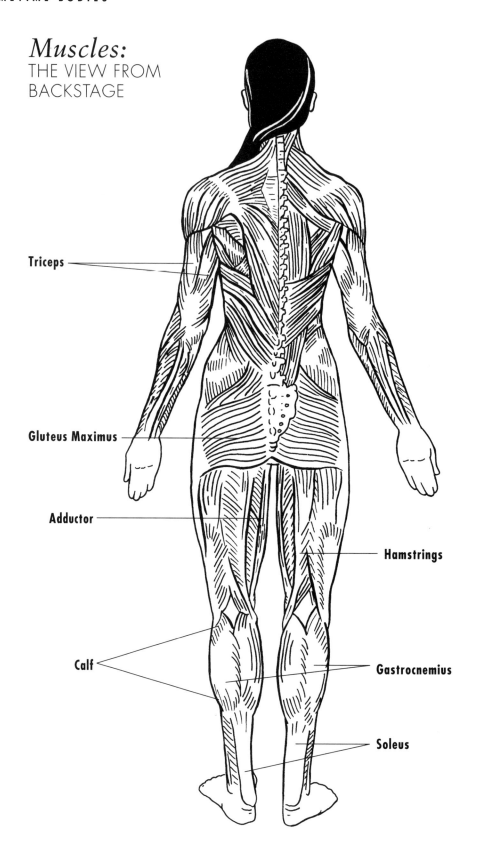

Triceps

Gluteus Maximus

Adductor

Hamstrings

Calf

Gastrocnemius

Soleus

toralis muscles help your breast area look more shapely.

BICEPS On the front of your upper arm, these muscles flex the upper arm. They're used to pull things toward you. When these muscles are strengthened they give your upper arm a shapelier look. Their opposing muscles are the triceps.

TRICEPS The muscles on the back of the upper arm. They act to extend the arm and forearm. The triceps tend to get flabby on women as we age. But we have some exercises that will help remedy that.

ABDOMINALS The rectus abdominis is a long powerful muscle that runs from your chest to your pubic bone. It pulls your torso toward your hips and your hips toward your torso. We'll work the "abs" with sit-ups, crunches, and leg raises.

OBLIQUES These muscles connect at the front half of the hip and the top of the pubis. The external obliques fuse with the fibrous tissue covering the rectus abdominis. The internal and external obliques rotate the trunk of your body and help you flex your torso. When we're down on the floor, we'll concentrate on the obliques with different moves in the sit-ups and crunches.

TRANSVERSE ABDOMINIS This muscle runs across the abdominals, underneath the external and internal obliques.

GLUTEUS MAXIMUS The large muscle that extends and rotates the thigh to the side. The "gluts" tend to drop on women, but our lunges and leg raises will give you a lift.

QUADRICEPS The front of the thigh. It's a group of four muscles that run down the front of the thigh to attach at the kneecap. These muscles all work to extend the leg and to flex the thigh. We'll work the "quads" when we do lunges, pliés, and leg extensions.

HAMSTRINGS Three muscles in the back of the thigh which flex the knee, rotate the leg, and extend the hips. We'll work the hamstrings both in a standing position and when we're on the floor working our gluts with leg raises.

ADDUCTOR These are the inner thigh muscles. They start at the pubic bone and go down to the side of the knee. They flex the thigh and pull the leg in toward the body.

ABDUCTOR—GLUTEUS MEDIUS While *abduction* is a movement away from the body, the term *abductor* is often confused with the outer thigh. Here *abductor* is used in conjunction with the gluteus medius, a short, thick muscle located above the gluteus maximus. It gives the rounded contour to the side of the hip.

CALF The muscle that runs from the knee to the ankle. It's important for the strength of the leg, and for women it's the part of the leg that is most often exposed. We'll be doing calf raises to strengthen the muscle and calf stretches to lengthen it.

GASTROCNEMIUS A superficial muscle that forms most of the calf. You'll work it in our calf raises.

SOLEUS The broad flat muscle just below the gastrocnemius. You'll stretch this muscle when you put your heel down in the calf stretch.

Now that you know the parts and you know the script, it's time to take the next step toward our performance. But before we do, let's look at our director—the person who will be calling the shots—you.

Shakespeare wrote "All the world's a stage and all the men and women merely players" (*As You Like It*). Going into the 21st century those words ring as true as ever. You may read about and admire the players you see on television and in movies, but remember—you've got your own program to appear in every day. You can look every bit as good playing your part as they do playing theirs.

Everyone has some body part she feels is her weakest, that she wants to work hardest to reduce, shape, and tone. For Claudia Schiffer it was shaping her thighs, for Melanie Griffith it was reducing and strengthening her "abs," for Jamie Gertz it was strengthening her legs, and for Penelope Ann Miller it was reducing and shaping her hips and outer thighs. For you it could be any single part or a combination of body parts that you want to work on.

As the director of your show, it's up to you to decide where you want to focus your workouts. Our six-week program puts all body parts in the spotlight.

3

Breathing Life into Your Performance

The Dramatic Effects

Actors know that one of the keys to portraying a character is getting the physicality of that character. Holly Hunter, for example, in her Academy Award–winning performance in *The Piano*, plays a mute but communicates exceptionally well with her eyes, with a turn of her head, with her body moving to include people she likes and to repel people she does not. And in *Terminator*, Linda Hamilton's show of strength and maneuverability tells how important it is for her to save herself and her son from danger. She definitely looks the part.

In order to deliver a great performance the actor must be in complete control of her body and so she must know how to make it act long before the director calls "action." And nothing is more important to good body condition and control than correct breathing.

Breathing is at the core of every actor's performance. It affects her posture, it affects her voice and speech, it affects her energy level, as well as the way she looks. Breathing is also central to effective exercise. You might find it hard to believe, but most people don't breathe correctly, because correct breathing, while it looks easy, takes work. It's like an actor giving a great performance . . . it looks effortless, but that's because of training, fine tuning, and lots of rehearsing.

We all know we must breathe in order to live. Oxygen keeps muscles and body tissues alive and healthy. If we want to burn off fat, we turn to activities that make us breathe harder and deeper because fat requires oxygen to burn. Aerobic activities such as walking, running, bicycling, and hiking are the most effective way to take off weight because they work your cardiovascular system at a high intensity, forcing your body to burn away fat. The benefits of aerobic exercise continue when oxygen is converted into energy, which raises your metabolism even after you've finished exercising, thereby keeping up the potential for fat burn-off.

Your abdominal area is the center of your body; it's not just geographically central—it's the center of your being. The abdominal muscles form a protective support for your vital internal organs. The abdominal area is where digestion and gestation take place. It's the part of the body from which you bend. Your abdominal muscles help support your lower back. It's also the place you will work with every breath you take throughout our six-week program.

Actually, you can get a workout just by breathing—if you're using your abdominal muscles in the right way. As you read this, you're probably sitting. Don't move. Just breathe in deeply through your nose. Now, as you blow out, blow out through your mouth and contract (pull in)

your stomach muscles. Do you feel your abdominals tightening? Slowly repeat this deep breathing in and out, making sure you contract your abdominals on the exhalation. Even if you feel your abs tightening up just a little, you're already on your way to a primetime body because you're strengthening your abs just by breathing!

When you exercise, it is best if you breathe out or exhale on the exertion. This exhalation contracts your stomach muscles and both draws strength from them and strengthens them.

We'll emphasize this breathing technique heavily during the abdominal sections of our workout but *this method of breathing should be used during all exercises* (particularly in aerobic exercises when most people don't give a lot of thought to the way they're breathing). Many people have a tendency to push out on their abs when they're exerting energy. That kind of breathing can only encourage a further protruding stomach area. That's because they're training their muscles the wrong way.

While you train yourself to breathe properly, your conscious efforts will pay off in some not-so-conscious ways. You'll find that as you practice controlled breathing in your exercises, your new way of breathing will become more the norm. And as your abs get stronger and flatter your posture will improve, which in turn will make you look longer and slimmer.

Nine out of ten women say they want flatter tummies. Breathing right during exercise will strengthen your abs and help flatten them. In addition, stronger abs will help protect your lower back. That means less chance for the common lower back pain so many people get.

There are other big benefits from strengthening your abs through breathing and exercise. Recent studies indicate that a strong and lean abdomen could help prevent heart disease. It seems that people who accumulate fat around their middles are more prone to heart attacks.

Weak abdominals are connected with prolapsed uterus, particularly (but not only) after childbirth when the abdominal muscles have been stretched excessively. Later in life, as muscle tone drops and belly muscles weaken, women are higher risk candidates for incontinence and again, prolapsed uterus. But the risk for both of these conditions is minimized with the right exercises that strengthen and tone the abdominals. Strong abs keep the pelvis in better alignment which in turn keeps the uterus, bladder, and intestinal tract in their proper place.

There's yet another major advantage to effective breathing—getting that oxygen flowing into your different body parts. The increased oxygen flow will stimulate your skin and help rid your skin of impurities. While the increased blood flow to your face carries that nutritious oxygen, your own sweat glands are providing moisture to your face that's even more valuable than anything that comes in a jar.

ONE LAST BREATH

Have you ever been so nervous the only way you could calm down was to breathe deeply? Actors use deep breathing to center themselves before a performance. They study relaxation techniques that use deep breathing as a way of relaxing their muscles and minds so they can be freer to take on the demands their characters place on them.

You'll find that breathing deeply will become your way of preparing for your own roles in life, whether they're in daily activities or when you have to face difficult times of stress.

Many clients, from Julianne Phillips to Tom Arnold, tell us that exercise gives them the mental stability they need to deal with stress. Penelope Ann Miller says that exercising regularly has helped her self-confidence and has definitely helped her career.

If these primetime bodies can do it, so can you. Take a deep breath now and let's get ready for our first workout.

4

Variety—It's Your Show

Week 1: The Body Parts Rundown

As the director calling the shots, you need to know what's on the program, where it appears, how long each segment will take, and how all the segments fit together. This is your "rundown."

Our primetime bodies rundown will change a bit each week of the program. We'll keep the basic elements all six weeks but we will also add on and modify moves as we go along. The changes will be based on your increasing endurance level. We will add some new twists to keep you interested in the plot and challenged enough to see it through.

Both the warm-up routine and the cool-down stretches will never change position in the rundown. We've given you a warm-up that will get your muscles warm and elevate your heart rate. Always warm up before you start *any* exercise routine. The warm-up will lessen your chance for injury because warm muscles are more flexible than cold ones. A cold start doesn't give you a chance to ease into character.

Even if an actor has done her research and prepared her own history of the character she is playing, and even if she has created a life for her character, it still takes time to get into character before a performance.

Your workout is your performance, and your warm-up is the prep time your character needs to perform at primetime levels. It's a psychological step as much as a physical one. Warm-up time is a good time to clear your mind of everything except the role you're about to perform. Warm-up and exercise time is your time to focus on yourself. You'll find that your workout will center you for the rest of your day.

You can decide how much time you want to give to your warm-up. We've designed a warm-up that will take about eight minutes. It will adequately prepare you for our routine, but we recommend at least 20 minutes of an additional aerobic activity. The benefits are big. First, it helps burn calories and that means burning off fat that covers the muscles we're going to help you shape. Second, it increases your metabolism even after you've finished this heart pumping activity, and that again means more efficient burning of calories (see Chapter 2). And aerobic activity improves your heart's health by helping to lower your blood pressure and cholesterol level. It also improves your lungs and respiratory system.

Aerobic activities use large muscle groups in rhythmic fashion for sustained periods of time. Some good aerobic exercises are bicycling, walking, running, swimming, hiking, and step classes. Or you can be creative: turn on your favorite Pointer Sisters album and dance around your living room for 15 to 20 minutes. Mix up your dancing with marching and jumping jacks.

Eventually you can work your way up to a 60-minute aerobic workout that you can do before you get into our program of shaping and toning your muscles. But no matter how much time you spend doing aerobics, try to do it at least four times a week for maximum results.

If you find that you don't have the extra time to do an aerobics workout in addition to our program, use our warm-up to prepare you for our program. But do it! You've got to make working out part of your schedule, and if you start missing those appointments with yourself it will be easy to get your whole program canceled. We'd rather see you get high ratings and stay up there with the best prime-time bodies.

BACKGROUND

Turn on some music. Just as any movie you watch uses music to inspire and create moods and add excitement to the action, you too should choose music that will drive your rhythms and will keep your spirits lifted as you go through our program.* Let's begin with our warm-up routine.

---

* We suggest music that has 110 to 120 beats per minute. Some recommendations: Janet Jackson, "Rhythm Nation"; Michael Jackson, "Bad"; Madonna, "Like a Virgin" or any albums by: Salt N Pepa, Bobby Brown, Gloria Estefan, Boyz II Men, or Dee-lite.

Action!

The Warm-Up

We'll start with getting your body moving and your blood circulating. Stand with your legs slightly more than shoulder-width apart and knees slightly bent. This is the basic position. Keeping your knees slightly bent supports your lower back. We'll be using this basic position throughout our program.

For each exercise, we give the number of repetitions (reps) we recommend as well as the number of "sets" of repetitions. If we say, for example, "Do 3 sets of 8 reps," you will do 24 total reps. If we say, "Do 2 sets of 10 reps," you will do 20 reps. A summary of the exercise rundown for each week, as well as for the warm-up and cool-down, appears at the end of each segment. These summaries list the number of reps and sets we recommend for each exercise.

Tap and Stretch

Reach your left arm up over your head and tap your left foot out to the side. Feel the stretch from your waist on your left side as you point your fingers up toward the ceiling. Now switch sides. As you tap your right foot out to the side, lift your right arm up and stretch it so your arm goes over your head and your fingers point up.

Each time you complete the tap and stretch on both sides is 1 repetition. Do 8 reps of this tap and stretch to complete 1 set. Do 2 sets.

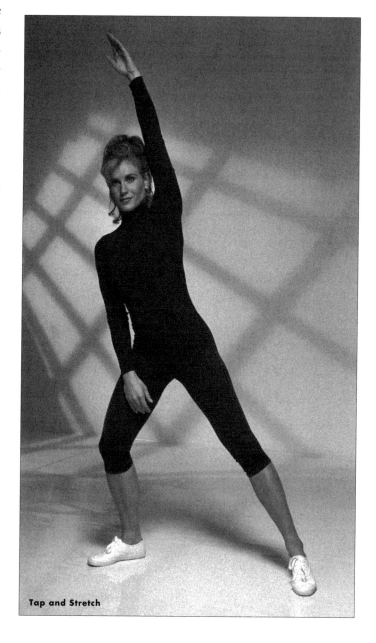

Tap and Stretch

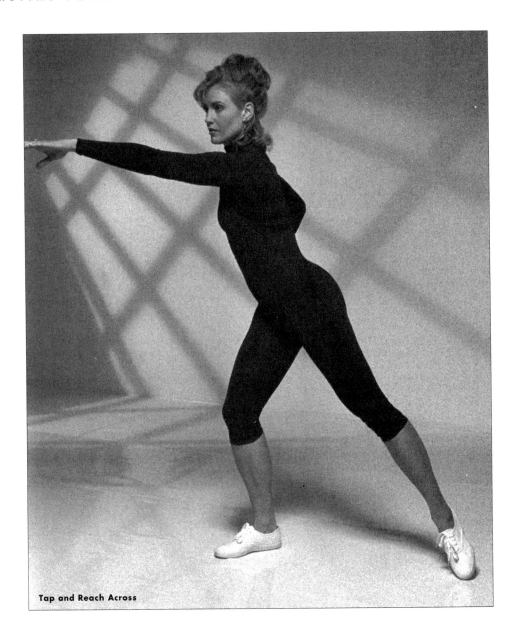

Tap and Reach Across

Tap and Reach Across

Change the upper body motion on this one so your left arm reaches across your chest at shoulder level while your left foot taps out to the side. You'll feel the stretch across your shoulders and waist on this one. Now switch sides and reach your right arm across your chest as you tap to the side with your right foot.

Each time you complete the tap and reach across on both sides is 1 rep. Do 2 sets of 8 reps.

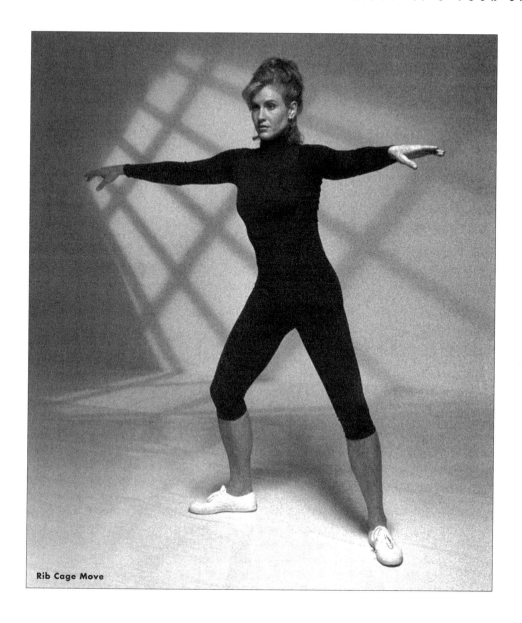

Rib Cage Move

Rib Cage Move

Get into the basic position, with your legs slightly more than shoulder-width apart, your knees slightly bent, and your toes turned out. Reach your arms out to the side and move your rib cage from right to left and then back to right. Remember to keep your arms at shoulder level and keep your lower body still while your upper body moves from the waist.

Each time you complete the move from right to left and back to right is 1 repetition. Do 2 sets of 8 reps.

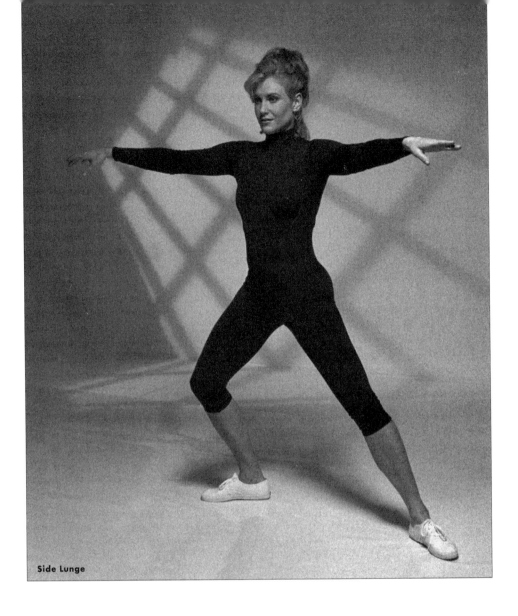

Side Lunge

Side Lunge

Keep your body in the same starting position as it was for the Rib Cage Move. You're going to work your legs and butt a little harder this time. Keep your upper body steady as you bend your right knee first. Bend it a little deeper than you did for the Rib Cage Move, stretching the inner thigh of your left leg which is angled straight out to your left side, making sure your knee is over your toe.

Hold this lunge position for a count of 8.

Then straighten your right leg as you bend your left knee, shifting your weight onto the left leg and stretching the inside of your right thigh. Hold for a count of 8.

Each time you complete the lunge on the right and left sides is 1 rep. Do 1 set of 8 reps.

Side Lunge Stretch

Still in the basic starting position, bend your right knee while you're holding your left leg out to the side and reach with your left arm up and over your head so that you're stretching from your waist at the same time you're stretching the left inner thigh and working your right quadriceps. Hold the stretch for a count of 8.

Switch sides and this time bend your left knee a little deeper while you reach over your head with your right arm. Hold for a count of 8.

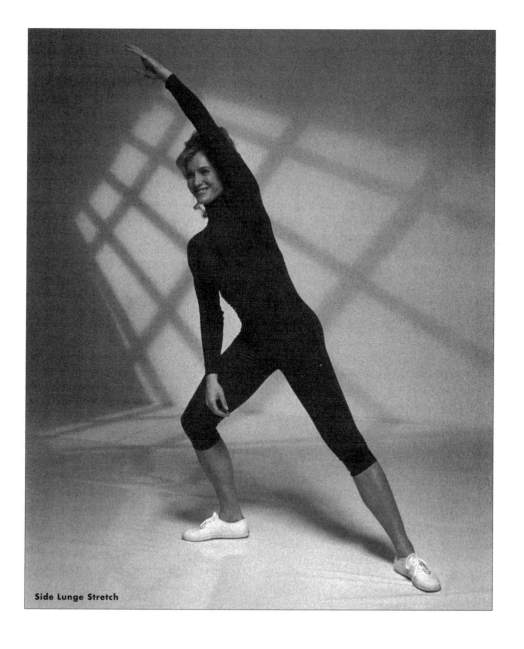

Side Lunge Stretch

Pliés

Stand with your hands on your waist, your feet slightly more than shoulder-width apart, and your knees and toes pointed out to the 10 and 2 positions on an imaginary clock. Keep your eyes focused straight ahead.

Now bend your knees and lower your body until you feel the stretch in your inner thighs. Always make sure your knees are pointed directly over your toes. Then lift and lower again, all the time squeezing your gluts.

Each time you lower and lift is 1 rep. Do 2 sets of 8 reps each.

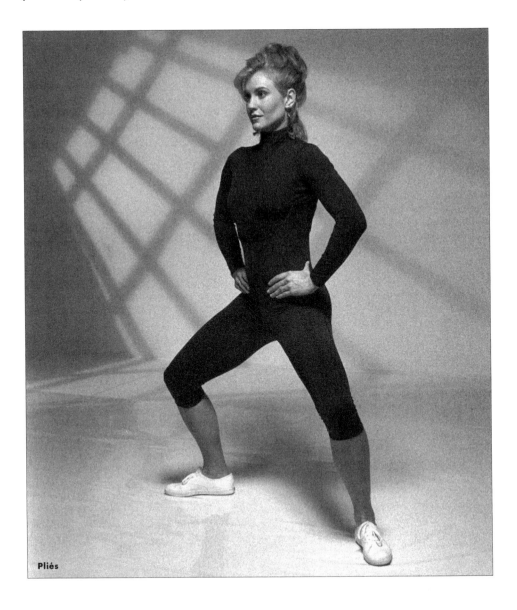

Pliés

Plié Heel Raise

You're still in the position for starting pliés. Now lift your right heel off the floor while your left foot remains flat and steady on the floor. Keeping your right heel raised, lower your body until you feel the stretch in your inner thighs. You'll feel your calf muscles working, too. Be careful to never let your knee extend farther than your toes. Now lift your body up.

Do 10 reps with your right heel raised and then 10 reps with your left heel raised.

Finish with both heels flat on the floor.

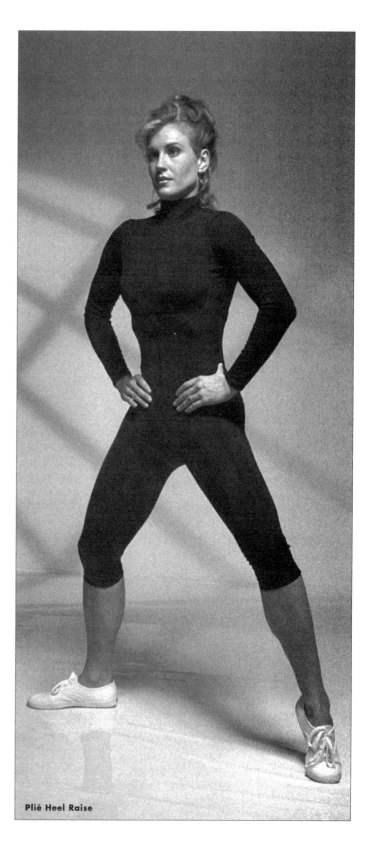

Plié Heel Raise

Lunges in Place

Turn to your right side and step your right leg forward and your left leg back. Your left heel is raised. Now balance yourself with your arms out in front of you at shoulder level as you lower your left knee to the floor. Do not rest your knee on the floor.

Your weight is on your right leg, working your quads and the right side of your butt. At the same time you will feel a stretch in the front of the left quad. Your knee must be in line with your ankle and should not bend farther forward than that.

You'll work your quad most effectively if you put your weight on your front leg and balance by using the ball of the back foot. Lift back into the starting position.

Now switch by stepping your left leg forward and your right leg back. Your right heel is raised. Using your arms stretched forward for balance, lower your right knee toward the floor. Make sure your front knee remains in line with your ankle. Lift back into starting position and start all over again with the right leg forward.

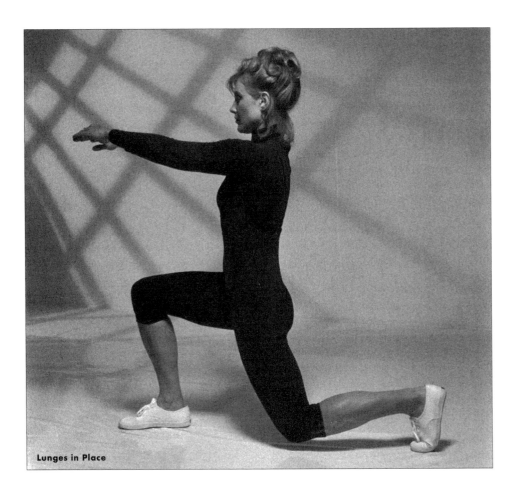

Lunges in Place

Do a total of 10 lunges on your right leg and 10 on your left.

At this point we want to do a few isolated stretches before we start moving around.

Calf Stretch

Bring your right leg forward, bent at the knee. Lift your left leg and extend it back comfortably with your heel raised. Now, keeping your leg straight, press your heel against the floor and hold it for 8 counts. You'll feel that stretch up and down your calf.

Alternate legs. Bring your left leg forward with your foot flat on the floor and knee slightly bent. Lift your right leg and extend it back with your heel raised. Now press your right heel down on the floor and hold this stretch for 8 counts. Stay where you are.

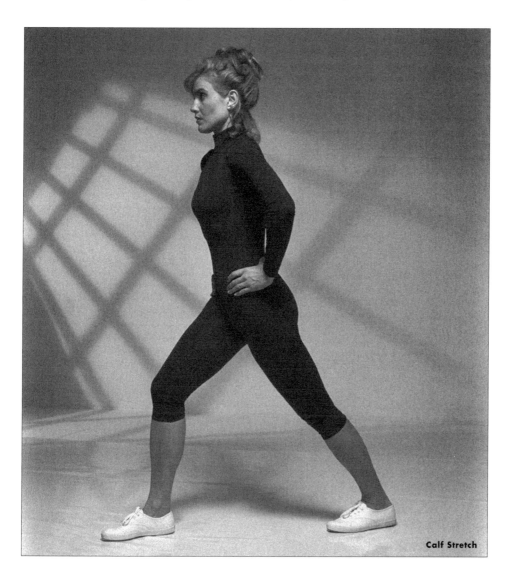

Calf Stretch

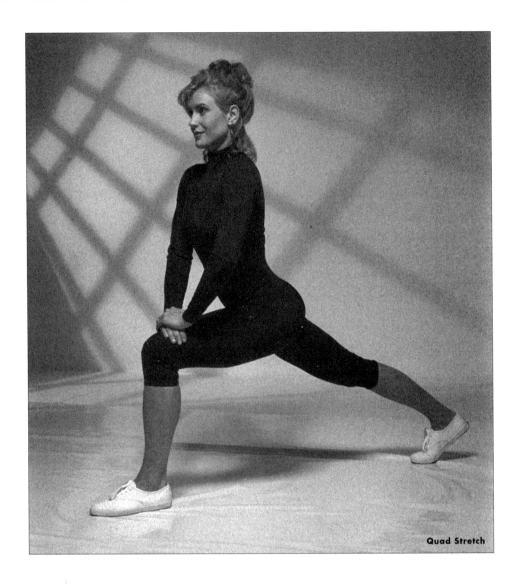

Quad Stretch

Quad Stretch

With your left leg forward and bent at the knee so your knee is aligned over your ankle, lift your right leg and take it back farther than it was for the calf stretch. Lift your right heel off the floor as you stretch the front of your right leg from your hip to your knee. Place your hands on your front leg for balance as you hold this quad stretch for 8 counts.

Now switch legs. Bring your right leg forward and bend it at the knee so it's at a right angle with the floor. Lift your left leg and place it as far back as comfortable. Lift your left heel off the floor as you stretch your left quad and hold it for a count of 8.

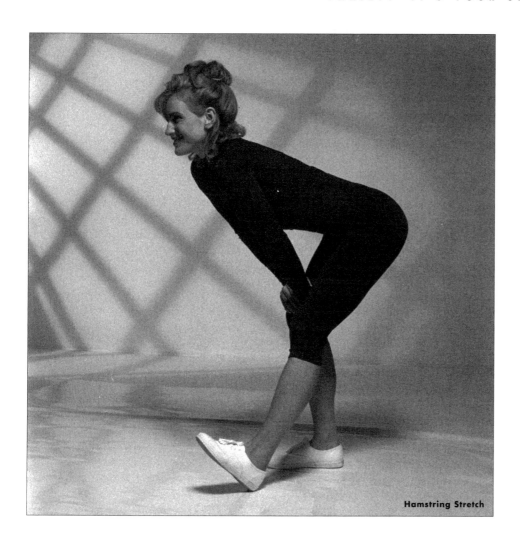

Hamstring Stretch

Hamstring Stretch

Place your left leg straight out in front of you, keeping your knee slightly bent and your toes pointed up. Your right leg is your support leg and, for balance, place your hands just above your slightly bent knee as you lean your upper body forward, stretching the hamstrings on your left leg. Hold the stretch for a count of 8.

Switch by placing your right leg straight out in front of you but keeping your knee slightly bent and your toes turned up. Your left leg, also with knee slightly bent, is now your support leg, and when you lean forward and extend your upper body over your extended leg, support yourself by resting your hands on your left leg. Hold the stretch for 8 counts.

Return to your original standing position and get ready to increase your heart rate.

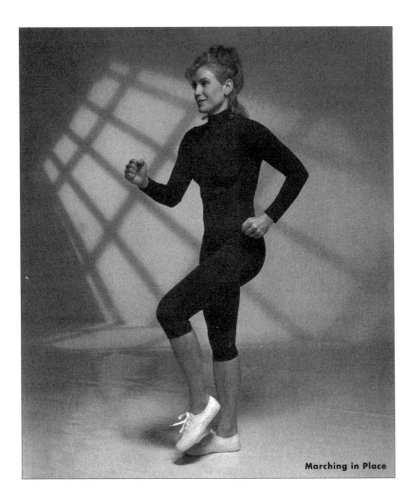

Marching in Place

Marching in Place

March in place by lifting your feet alternately at least a couple of inches off the floor while you swing your bent arms forward and back. Don't forget to breathe deeply. Exhale as you lift and lower one foot and inhale as you lift and lower the other foot.

Count each pair of lifts of the right and left leg as 1 rep. March 4 sets of 8 reps.

Elbow-to-Knee March

Take the march down to half time, lifting your knees waist high or higher as you cross your right elbow to your left uplifted knee followed by your left elbow to your right uplifted knee. Breathe out each time you lift your bent knee to touch your elbow.

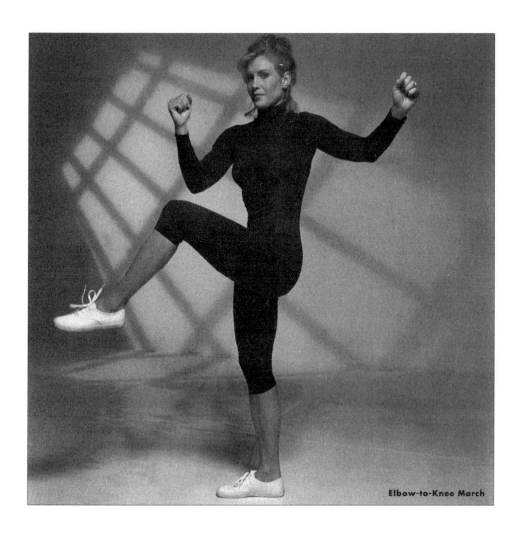

Elbow-to-Knee March

Count each pair of leg lifts with the opposite elbow touch as 1 rep.

March 2 sets of 8 reps.

Marching in Place

Again with your knees bent, lift your feet off the floor as you swing your bent arms back and forth. Remember to breathe steadily, exhaling when you lift and inhaling when you lower.

Do 4 sets of 8 reps.

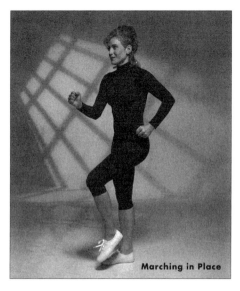

Marching in Place

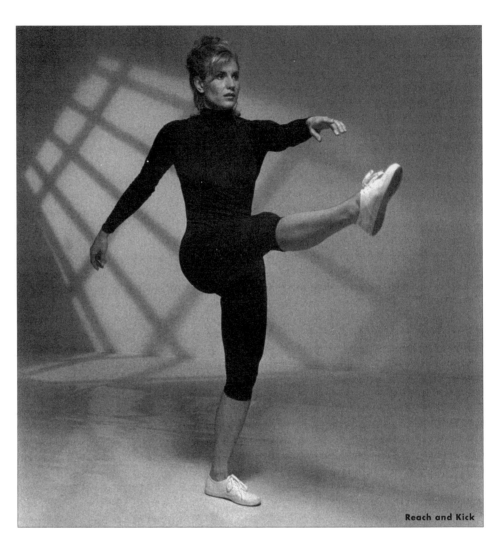

Reach and Kick

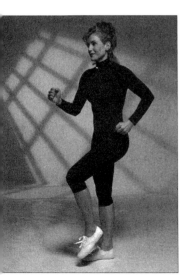

Reach and Kick

Kick your right leg forward and up at least waist high while you reach toward your pointed toes with the left arm. Then kick your left leg forward and up at least waist high while you reach your right arm forward toward your pointed toes. Exhale on the lift of the leg and inhale as you set the leg down.

Do 2 sets of 8 reps.

Marching in Place

Repeat the march in place by lifting your feet off the floor, knees bent, as you swing your arms back and forth.

Do 2 sets of 8 reps.

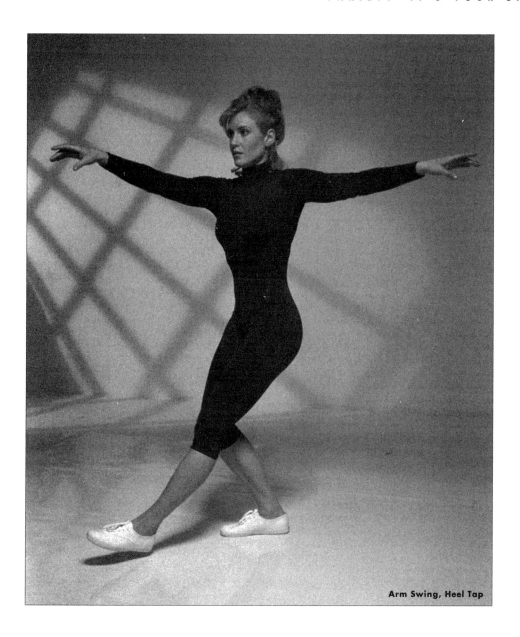

Arm Swing, Heel Tap

Arm Swing, Heel Tap

Swing your arms forward and back at your sides, while you extend your right foot forward and tap your right heel on the floor in front of you. Then as you continue swinging your arms, bring your right leg back to starting position as you bring your left leg forward, foot flexed, heel tapping the floor as your opposite arm swings forward.

Count each heel tap of the right foot and left foot as 1 rep. Do 2 sets of 8 reps.

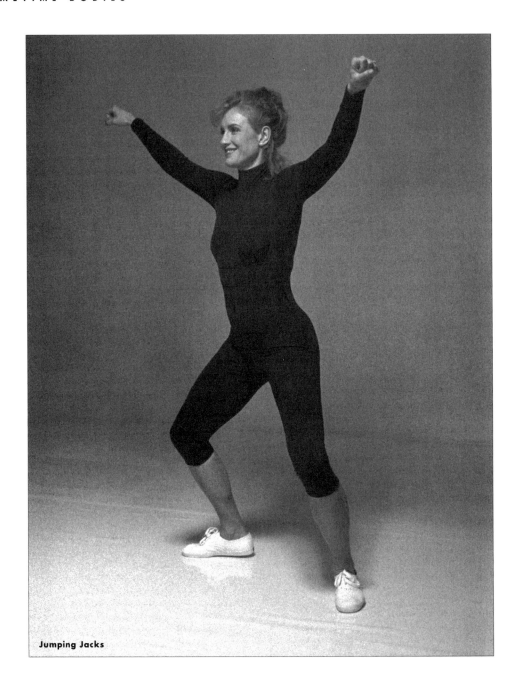

Jumping Jacks

Jumping Jacks

Get into the basic position. Starting with your hands at your sides, use the balls of your feet to spring your legs out to the side while your arms swing up to meet overhead. As you bring your arms down, your legs jump back to starting position.

Do 1 set of 10 jumping jacks. If you find jumping uncomfortable, try the following exercise.

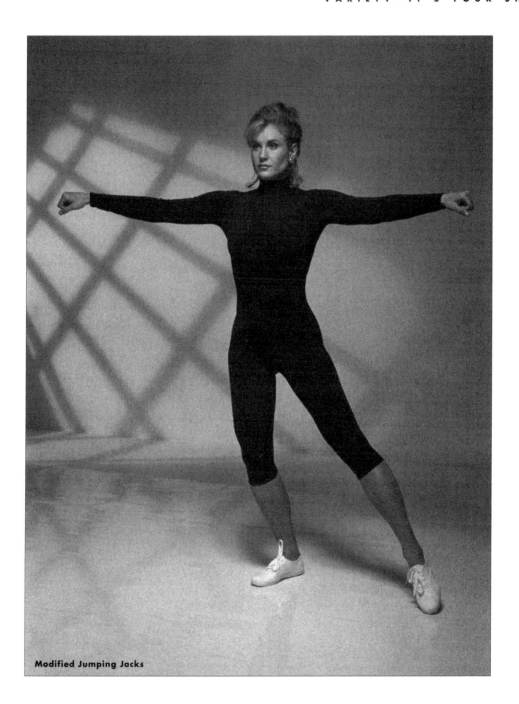

Modified Jumping Jacks

Modified Jumping Jacks

While you lift your arms out to the side and up to shoulder level, first take your right leg out to the side with your toe pointed to the floor. As your arms come back down to your side, bring the right foot in and move your left leg out to the side.

Do 1 set of 10 reps.

Arm Swing, Heel Tap

Swing your arms forward and back at your sides while you extend your right leg forward, tapping your right heel. Then bring your left leg forward, tapping your left heel.

Do 2 sets of 8 reps.

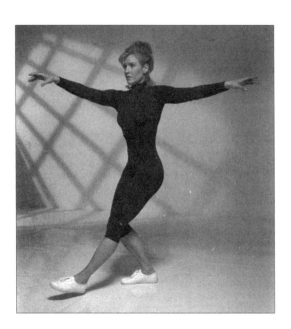

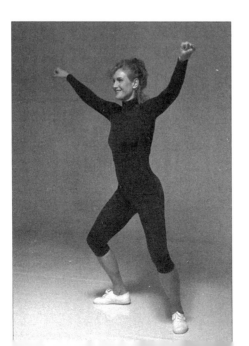

Jumping Jacks

Start with your legs shoulder-width apart and your knees bent. Push off your feet to jump your legs out to the sides while you swing your arms up and over your head. As your arms come back down to your sides, jump back to starting position.

Do 1 set of 10 Jumping Jacks. Or you may substitute with Modified Jumping Jacks.

March in Place

With bent knees, lift each foot alternately, at least a couple of inches off the floor as you swing your arms back and forth.

Do 2 sets of 8 reps.

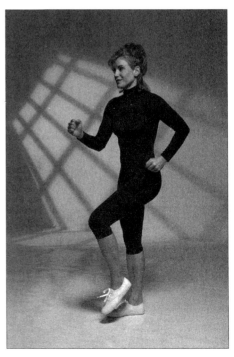

March in Place— Half Speed

March at half speed while you breathe deeply, inhaling and exhaling, focusing on your abs.

Do 1 set of 8 reps.

Head and Neck Roll

Standing in the basic position, let's loosen your neck and shoulders. First, gently stretch the left side of your neck by tilting your head to your right, pointing your right ear toward your right shoulder. Hold for a count of 10.

Then gently roll your head forward so that your chin reaches down toward your chest. Hold for a count of 10.

Now slowly roll your head over to your left side as you gently stretch the right side of your neck. Hold for a count of 10.

At this point, you should be feeling warmed up and your heart rate should be elevated. Now the curtain is going up and it's time to start unveiling those muscles. . . .

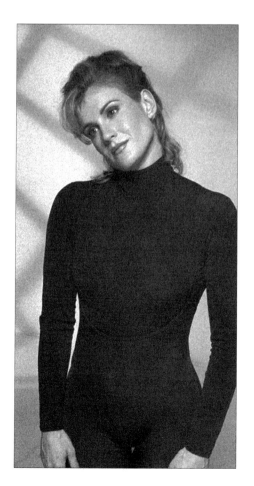
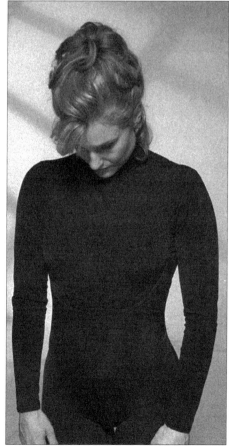

WARM-UP SUMMARY

Exercise	Reps Per Set	Sets
Tap and Stretch	8	2
Tap and Reach Across	8	2
Rib Cage Move	8	2
Side Lunge	8	1
Side Lunge Stretch	hold 8 counts each side	
Pliés	8	2
Plié Heel Raise	10 right/10 left	
Lunges in Place	10 right/10 left	
Calf Stretch	hold 8 counts each side	
Quad Stretch	hold 8 counts each side	
Hamstring Stretch	hold 8 counts each side	
March in Place	8	4
Elbow-to-Knee March	8	2
March in Place	8	4
Reach and Kick	8	2
March in Place	8	2
Arm Swing, Heel Tap	8	2
Jumping Jacks (or Modified Jumping Jacks)	10	1
Arm Swing, Heel Tap	8	2
Jumping Jacks	10	1
March in Place	8	2
March in Place—Half Speed	8	1
Head and Neck Roll	hold 10 counts each, right, front, left	

Week 1

Overhead Press

Stand in the basic position with your legs apart and knees slightly bent, keeping the pelvis neutral (not tilted forward or backward). Start with your arms lifted at your side, bent at the elbow with your hands in a loose fist facing forward.

Now raise your arms and exhale, straightening them until they're fully extended overhead, as if you're pressing up to the ceiling. Hold for a beat; then inhale as you return your arms to their original position.

Complete 1 set of 10 reps.

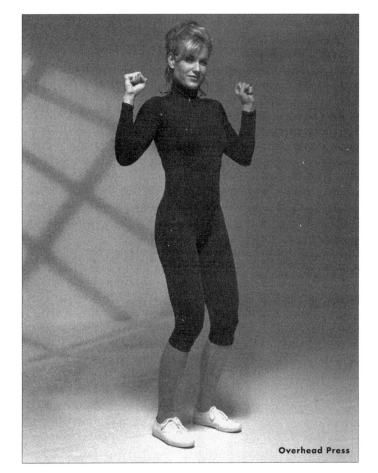

Overhead Press

Rear Deltoids

Sit at the edge of your chair and bend forward at the waist with your arms down at your sides. Lift your arms out to the sides and bring them up to shoulder level. Squeeze your shoulder blades together and exhale, working your posterior deltoids, and return your arms to your sides.

Do not drop your head; keep it forward and aligned with your spine.

Complete 1 set of of 10 reps.

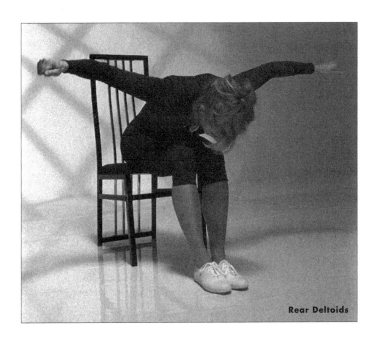

Rear Deltoids

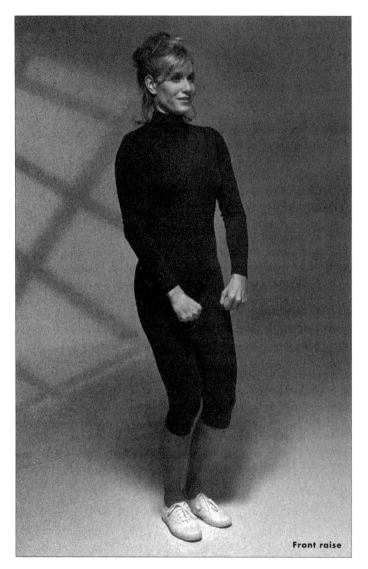

Front raise

Biceps Curls

You're still in your basic standing position with your arms at your sides. Turn your palms forward and make a loose fist. Now curl your arms up toward your shoulders so your fists face your shoulders at the top. Squeeze your biceps as you curl up, and when you return your arms to the starting position, resist the movement as if there were a heavy weight in your hands. (In later weeks we'll be adding weights to many of our exercises.)

Do not turn your wrists. Keep them steady with your palms facing up throughout the entire movement.

Do 3 sets of 10 reps.

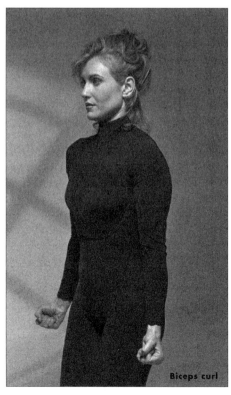

Biceps curl

Front Raise

In the basic position, with feet just slightly apart and your hands in loose fists, palm side down, take a deep breath and begin to exhale as you lift both arms in front of you to shoulder height. Then, taking another deep breath, return your arms to the original position.

Complete 1 set of 10 reps.

Triceps Extension

We'll work your right arm first. Standing on your right leg, place your left knee on your chair and bend at the waist until your torso is extended over and parallel to the chair seat. Balance your upper body with your left arm and bring your right arm up, bending it at the elbow and making sure the top of your arm is parallel to your back. Relax your left knee to make sure your back is flat.

Now with your right hand in a loose fist that faces your body, extend your arm back, keeping the elbow level with the shoulder. Squeeze your triceps and then return to the starting position.

Repeat 10 times and then switch sides.

Turn so that your right knee is resting on the chair and your right arm is supporting your upper body. Plant your left foot on the floor and bend your upper body from the waist, until it's parallel to the chair seat. Put your left arm up and bent at the elbow, and your hand in a loose fist facing your body.

Now extend your left arm back so it is parallel to the floor. Squeeze the triceps and release; return to the starting bent-elbow position.

Repeat 10 times.

By working both arms 10 times each, you have just completed 1 set. Do 2 more (3 total) sets of 10 on each arm.

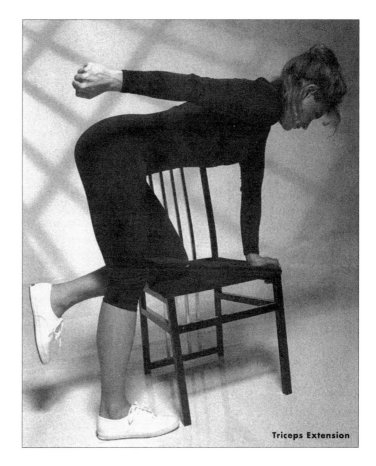

Triceps Extension

Now we'll move down to the lower body.

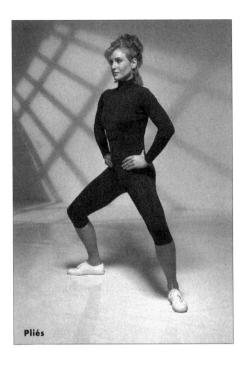

Pliés

Pliés with Pulses

Start with the regular plié down but when you're at the bottom, where your butt is almost at a 45-degree angle to your knee, pulse for 3 counts. "Pulse" means lift slightly and lower slightly so you feel the added work on your butt and your inner thighs.

Do 5 reps of the plié with a pulse at the bottom.

Pliés

Now do 5 regular pliés. You're ready to move on.

Pliés

Your basic plié position is with your legs more than shoulder-width apart and your toes pointed in the 10 and 2 positions on an imaginary clock.

With your hands on your hips, lower your body, bending your knees so that your torso comes toward the floor. As you go deeper toward the floor, your knees are over your toes. Your pelvis should stay neutral. Stop before your butt gets to a 45-degree angle to your knees. Your knees should be at a 45-degree angle to your ankles.

Now as you lift up, squeeze your gluts. Do not come all the way up to a straight leg because you want to keep the tension. Stop when your knees are slightly bent.

Repeat 5 times.

Hamstrings

You'll need your chair for this one. Facing the back of the chair, and resting forearms on it for support, walk your legs back a few steps from the chair. Stand on your left leg with your knee relaxed, your right leg bent slightly at the knee. Flex your right foot and bend your right leg more, squeezing as you bring your heel toward your butt.

Keep your pelvis neutral as you lift your bent leg up and place it down. Make sure you keep your knees together to help isolate your hamstring muscle.

Do this movement 8 times.

Now switch legs. Stand on your right leg and lift your left leg back

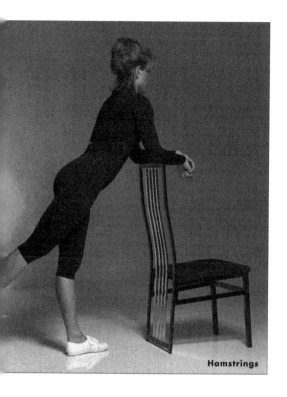

Hamstrings

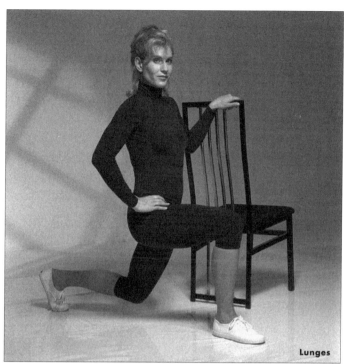

Lunges

and bend it slightly at the knee. Aim your left heel toward your butt as you squeeze your gluts. Now lower your leg back to the starting position.

Repeat this movement 8 times and get ready to take the:

Lunges

Turn to your right and stand next to the back of the chair. Holding on to it for support, bring your right leg forward and leave your left leg back. Raise your left heel and bend your left knee as you lower it toward the floor. Go down only as far as you can—but never touch the floor with your knee. Ultimately, your calf should end up parallel to the floor and your right leg should form a right angle from your hip to your knee and knee to foot. Never let your front knee come forward over your toes.

Hold the lunge position for a beat and then push up with your right leg, using the heel of your right foot to help push as you squeeze your butt on the way up. Lunges are great for your quads and your gluts.

This week we're starting with 8 lunges on your right leg.

Now switch legs. Bring your left leg forward, bending it at the knee so it forms a right angle, and at the same time lower your right knee toward the floor—go as low as you can without touching the floor. Hold for a beat and push up with the weight on your left heel.

Do 8 lunges on your left leg.

Calf Raises

We're going to strengthen and shape your calves with this exercise.

Holding on to the chair for balance, lift both your heels up, pressing forward onto your toes and then lower your heels back to the floor.

Repeat this up-and-down motion 10 times.

Calf Raises— Heels Together

Now put your heels together and lift your heels up by rolling your weight forward onto your toes. Do this 10 times.

Calf Raises— Toes Together

Change your foot position so that your toes are together and your heels are separated. Lift your heels off the floor by pushing your weight onto your toes.

Repeat this 10 times.

Toe Taps

Let's start strengthening your lower front leg—your shins—by tapping your toes.

Put your weight on your right leg and start tapping your left foot.

With your heel on the floor, raise the toes on your left foot as high as you can and bring them down, then up and down again. Do 10 reps with your left foot.

Now switch your weight onto your left leg as you tap your right foot 10 reps. Ten taps on each foot completes 1 set.

Repeat a second set of 10 taps with each foot.

Calf Stretch

If you did our warm-up, you've done this stretch once. Don't skip it; do it again. You need to stretch your calves after doing the Calf Raises and the Toe Taps.

Bring your right leg forward and bend it slightly at the knee. Extend

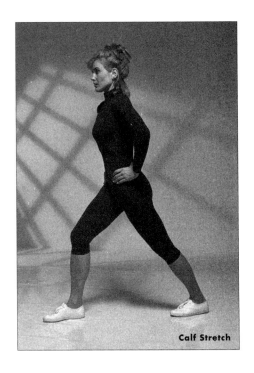

Calf Stretch

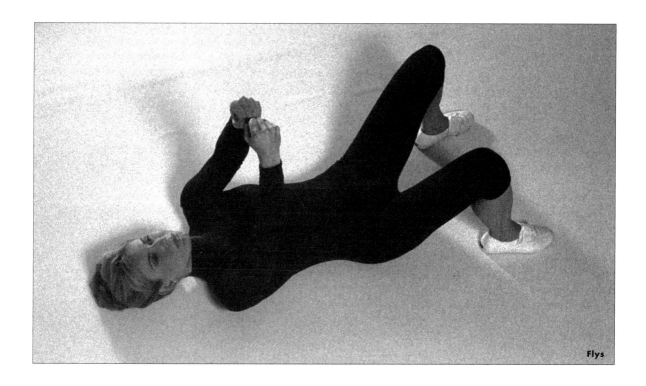

Flys

your left leg behind you, far enough so that your heel is raised. Gently press your left heel against the floor and stretch. Hold for a count of 8.

Now switch by bringing your left leg forward and bend it slightly at the knee. Extend your right leg behind you with your heel raised. Gently press your right heel against the floor and stretch your right calf. Hold for a count of 8.

Let's take to the floor for our next program segment.

Flys

Lie down on the floor on your back with your arms extended overhead. Bend your legs at the knees with your feet on the floor. This will pro-

tect your lower back as you work your chest and shoulders.

Lower your arms out to the sides, keeping your elbows slightly bent. Feel the stretch across your chest. Now exhale as you lift your arms back to the starting position. Do 3 sets of 10 reps.

Next is one of the best upper-body exercises there is.

Push-Ups

Roll over so you're lying on your stomach. Lift your body so your weight is on your extended arms and bent knees. Raise your feet and cross your ankles. Your hands, fingers facing forward, should be in line with your shoulders. Your head is forward, face looking down toward the floor.

Inhale as you lower your body. Keep your back straight and come down as far as you can without touching the floor. Tighten your abs with your exhalation and lift, squeezing your butt and keeping your pelvis in a neutral position. This should help you make sure that your back is straight. Now inhale and lower again toward the floor but do not rest on the floor. Lift again. When you get all the way back up, straighten your arms but do not lock your elbows.

Do 5 Push-Ups to complete 1 set.

You'll need a good stretch here. Push-ups really give the backs of your arms, your shoulders, and your chest a challenge. And if you continue to do the breathing right, you will be working your abs at the same time. So remain on the floor, lying on your stomach.

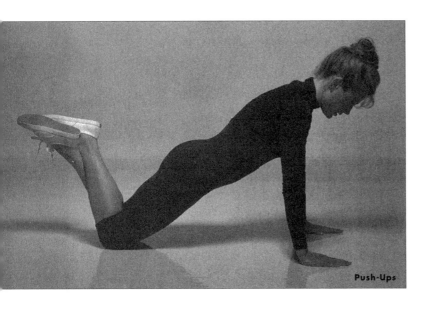

Push-Ups

Back Stretch

Lift your right arm and your left leg at the same time, exhaling as you lift. Make sure your left foot is flexed, with your toes pointing down. Stretch your arm and your leg as far as you can. Hold for a count of 8, breathing deeply as you hold.

Now switch so that your left arm and right leg are lifted and stretching. Exhale on the lift; hold and breathe deeply for a count of 8.

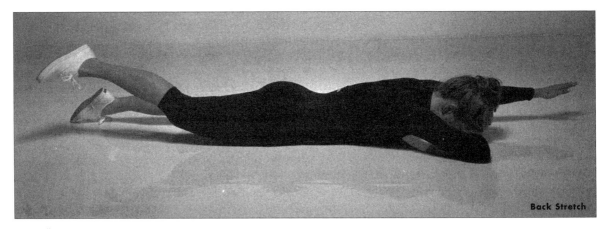

Back Stretch

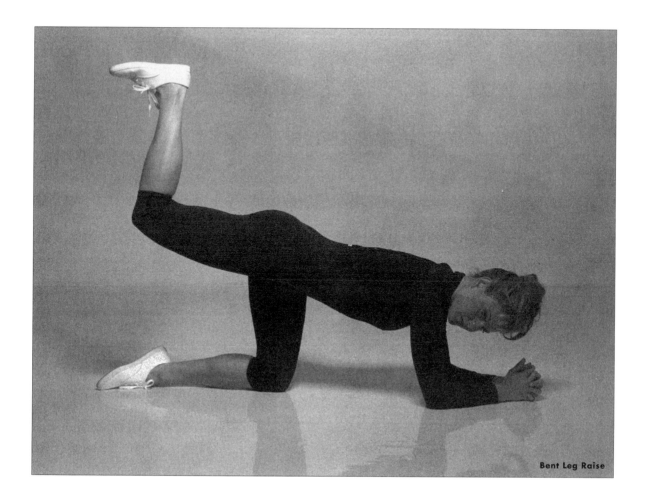

Bent Leg Raise

Bent Leg Raise

Now with your stretched-out arms and legs, push yourself up so that you're resting on your elbows and knees.

This one is for your hamstrings and gluts. Your knees are positioned right below your hips and your elbows are positioned below your shoulders with your hands out in front of you. Keep your back straight and pull your abs in toward your spine.

Now raise your right leg up, keeping your knee bent and your right foot flexed. Exhale on the lift, pulling in on your abs. Aim to bring your knee level with your butt, squeezing and isolating the hamstring and glut. Now inhale as you bring your working leg back to the original position. Repeat this move 8 times with the right leg.

Switch legs now, raising your left leg up so that you wind up with your left quad facing the floor and the sole of your left foot facing the ceiling. Remember to exhale on the lift and inhale when you bring your left leg back down to its original position. Repeat the move 8 times with your left leg.

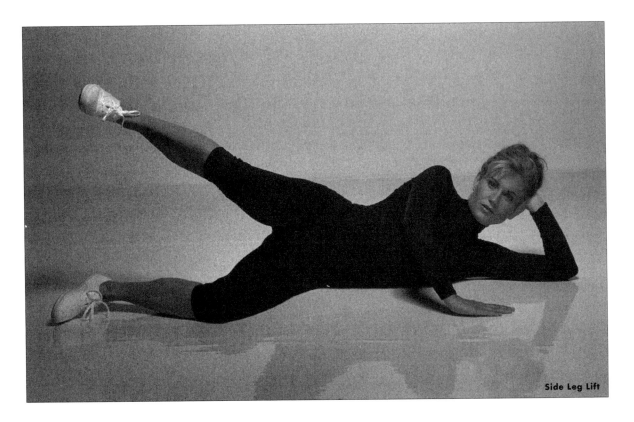

Side Leg Lift

Come down off your knees and lie down on your left side, ready to work your outer thigh muscles.

Side Leg Lift

Bend your knees at an angle to your hips of about halfway between 45 and 90 degrees. Your hips and legs are stacked so that the inside of your top knee (your right knee on this one) is looking down on the inside of your lower knee.

Rest your bottom arm—the left one—on the floor, bent at the elbow, and rest your head in that hand. Place your right arm out in front of your chest for support.

Now lift your top leg, but lift it only as high as you can without rolling backward. You must stay steady to keep the outer thigh working. When you lower your leg, squeeze your butt as you bring your leg down. Do not let your upper and lower legs touch before you lift your upper leg again.

Do 3 sets of 8 reps.

Turn onto your right side now, with your legs together and extended forward with your knees bent. Lift your left leg up so you can feel your gluts working. Remember to exhale when you lift so that your abs can help support your move. Now lower your leg and squeeze your butt at the same time you inhale.

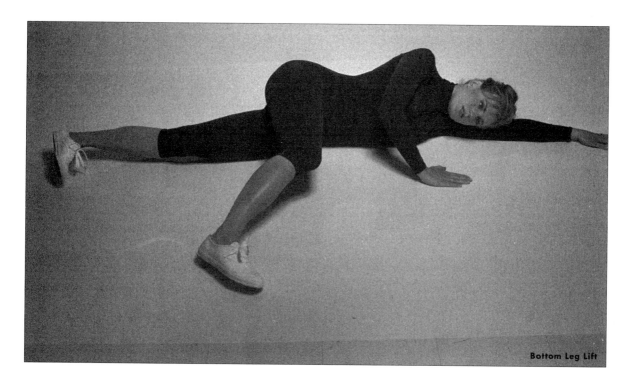

Bottom Leg Lift

Do 3 sets of 8 reps. Now let's work the adductors.

Bottom Leg Lift

This one works your inner thigh muscles—the adductors. Lying on your left side, your body is in a straight line. Rest your head on your outstretched lower arm and place your right arm in front of you for support. Bring your top leg over in front of you, keeping your hips stacked (aligned with your spine), and flex your bottom foot.

Now exhale as you lift your bottom (left) leg, and lower but do not let it touch the floor before you lift it again.

Do 3 sets of 8 reps.

Now turn over to work the other side. Lying on your right side with your legs together, extend the upper leg out in front of you. Rest your head on your right extended arm. Your right leg is in a straight line with your right arm.

As you exhale, lift your right leg, squeezing the inner thigh. Keep your foot flexed. Now lower the leg without touching the floor.

Do 3 sets of 8 reps.

Get ready to work those abs.

Abdominals

This first week will give you the basic abdominals workout. Each week, we'll change and add on to this section so that you will steadily get a more challenging workout.

We'll be working your entire abdominal area which, as you strengthen it, will help reduce your risk for lower back pain and improve your posture. But strengthening your abs won't get rid of fat in your abdominal area. We'll build up your muscle but if you are overweight, your toned muscle will remain hidden under whatever fat you may have.

If you need to lose weight, we suggest you follow a low-fat diet and count your calories. We also suggest you work at burning off your calories by challenging your body with aerobic exercise, as we mentioned at the beginning of this chapter.

We also want to stress the importance of drinking lots of water. It will keep you feeling full at the same time it helps you lose weight by flushing out your system. And when you're in an exercise session it will help replace the fluids your body loses during exercise.

So, it's time to take a few sips of water and get ready to make your middle your top priority for the last couple of minutes of your workout.

Crunches

Lie on the floor on your back. Bend your knees and place your feet flat on the floor in front of you. With your hands behind your head and your chin off your chest, lift your shoulders off the floor and up toward your knees.

(There are some things to be careful of here. One is that you don't pull on your head or neck to lift off the floor—use your abs to do that pulling. Another is that you keep your chin up, but not too high. Picture your chin holding a grapefruit resting on your chest. That's where your chin should be. And last, get your breathing right. Remember to exhale at the point of most exertion—so you exhale when you're lifting up and inhale when your torso goes back down.

Do this move 8 times up and down—counting each round-trip as 1—to complete 1 set.

Sit-Ups with Pulses

Repeat the same move but this time pulse 3 times when you get to the top of your lift and then lower back down. Do not let your upper back touch the floor.

Do 8 reps to complete 1 set.

Two-Count Crunches

Now change the move to 2 counts up and then 2 counts down. So you lift to about halfway up on the first count and then you lift again on the second count. Now take your upper body down halfway for the first count and the rest of the way on the second count. Make the move smooth but increase the intensity by doing it in 2 counts.

Do 8 reps to complete 1 set.

Crunches with Pulses

Now do 8 more reps with 3 pulses at the top of each lift.

Crunches

Come back down and then repeat the original move which is a curl up and a curl down.

Do 8 of these to complete the abs workout. And get ready for the cool-down stretch.

Cool-Down Stretches

You may be tempted to skip this last part of your workout, but don't give in. You're like the actress who has just finished her performance and left the stage. Your mind and body are still at your performance peak and even though you're looking forward to moving on, you're actually still in character. You need a cool-down so you can lower your heart rate and stretch the muscles you have worked.

These last stretches will keep you flexible and will help you avoid soreness. Stretching will help you avoid injuries to your muscles, too.

Consider your cool-down stretch your postproduction. It's the time you've got to wrap up the show.

WEEK 1 SUMMARY

Exercise	Reps	Sets
Overhead Press	10	1
Rear Deltoids	10	1
Front Raise	10	1
Biceps Curls	10	3
Triceps Extension	10 right/10 left	3
Pliés	5	1
Pliés with Pulses	5	1
Pliés	5	1
Hamstrings	8 right/8 left	1
Lunges	8 right/8 left	1
Calf Raises	10	1
Calf Raises—Heels Together	10	1
Calf Raises—Toes Together	10	1
Toe Taps	10 right/10 left	2
Calf Stretch	hold 8 counts each side	
Flys	10	3
Push-Ups	5	1
Back Stretch	hold 8 counts each side	
Bent Leg Raise	8 right/8 left	1
Side Leg Lift	8 right/8 left	3
Bottom Leg Lift	8 right/8 left	3
Crunches	8	1
Sit-Ups with Pulses	8	1
Two-Count Crunches	8	1
Crunches with Pulses	8	1
Crunches	8	1

Contract and Relax Whole Body

Still on the floor, flat on your back, extend your arms overhead and tighten your muscles from the tips of your fingers all the way down your body—down your arms, your abs, your gluts, your quads, your calves, your toes. Even squeeze your eyes shut. Hold your contraction for a count of 8, then relax.

Knees-to-Chest Stretch

Bend one knee and, using both hands placed on the underside of your thigh, pull it to your chest. Hold for a count of 10.

Release this leg and switch by bringing up your other bent leg and pull it into your chest. Hold for another count of 10.

Now bring up both knees and hold them into your chest for your last count of 10.

Hip-Glut Stretch

Bring your feet down and stretch your legs on the floor. Stretch your right arm straight out to the side, and bring your right knee to your chest and cross it over your left leg. Keep your right arm stretched out to the side while your left hand gently presses your right knee down to the floor.

Hold this stretch for a count of 10.

Switch sides by straightening your right leg and placing your left arm out to your side. Bend your left knee and bring it up over your right

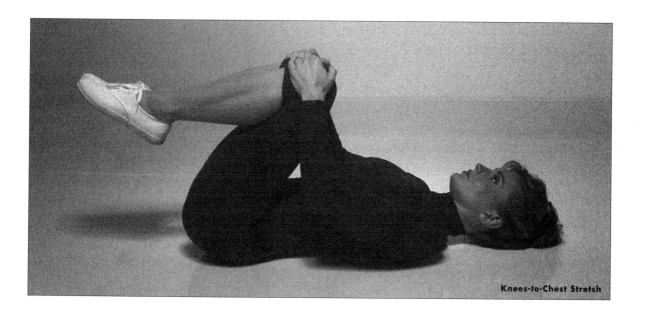

Knees-to-Chest Stretch

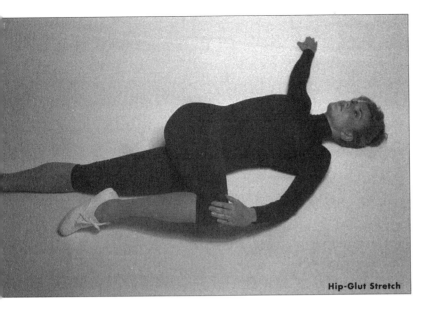

Hip-Glut Stretch

leg. Use your right hand to gently stretch your leg, pressing your knee to the floor.

Hold for a count of 10. Sit up to get into position for the:

Wide-Legged Stretch

Open your legs into a V position. Open only to a comfortable distance. Do not force this stretch. As the weeks go by you'll get more flexible and you'll find you'll be able to open your legs into a wider position.

So for now, with your legs open as far as is comfortable, reach your right arm up overhead and point your outstretched fingers toward your left flexed foot. At the same time, bend to your left side so that your left shoulder comes down toward your left knee and your left arm rests on the floor in front of your left quad. Your resting arm is bent at the elbow.

Hold this stretch for a count of 10.

Release and switch sides, stretching your left arm up over your head while your right shoulder goes down toward your right knee. Your right arm is in front of you for balance.

Hold the stretch for a count of 10. Release.

Bring your legs together. Now reach up with both hands overhead and clap them together.

You deserve the applause— you've just completed your workout and you're on your way to a primetime body.

COOL-DOWN STRETCHES SUMMARY

Exercise	Hold
Contract and Relax Whole Body	8 counts
Knees-to-Chest Stretch	10 counts, right, left, and both
Hip-Glut Stretch	10 counts, right and left
Wide-Legged Stretch	10 counts, right and left

5

Building on the Basics

Week 2: More Action

One of the primary reasons actors become actors is that they want to express themselves and they want validation. It's the reason Sally Field's statement "You like me, you really like me" got such a rousing reception from an audience full of actors at the Academy Awards ceremony in 1985, when she won an Oscar for her role in *Places in the Heart.*

Thousands of people dream of joining the acting ranks every year even though they may have only the desire and no training or even knowledge of how actors work. But if that desire is strong enough, training and imagination are the stepping stones to turning that dream into reality.

It's not all that different for you as you dream about getting yourself into great shape. Everyone wants the results, the compliments that go with a great figure, the self-satisfaction that comes with being the best that you can be.

It always looks easy from the outside, but any "overnight sensation" will tell you how many months or years of training it actually took and how much rejection she had to endure before she really made it. Because she believed in herself, she rose above the rest. Because she did what it took, she made it to where she wanted to go. She became a primetime body and so can you.

We have a story to illustrate the point. Penelope Ann Miller had already appeared in several major films when she auditioned for the lead opposite

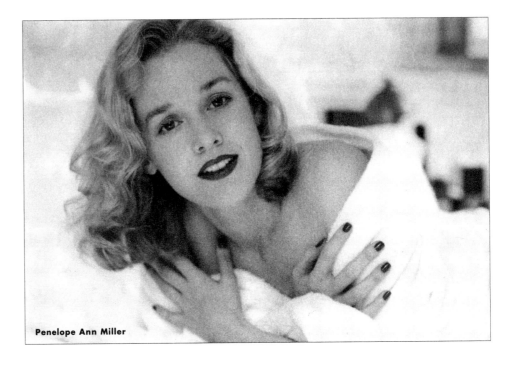

Penelope Ann Miller

Al Pacino in *Carlito's Way*. It was a great part and the chance to appear with one of the best actors in America.

Pacino liked the way Penelope read but she was only halfway there. You see, the part was that of a stripper and she had to look the part.

The next segment of her audition—a screen test—was to be three weeks later and she was to wear a bikini. We decided to exercise 18 out of the 21 days she had. We made a plan that included hiking the Santa Monica Mountains, step-and-slide, treadmill, biking, and more hiking.

We combined those aerobic activities with an accelerated version of the exercises in the program you're doing. We worked especially hard on Penelope's hips and thighs. And by the end of the three weeks, Penelope's legs looked firmer and slimmer, and improved muscle tone was apparent.

Penelope said she felt so much more confident about herself when she did the screen test that she could concentrate on her acting without being self-conscious about the way she looked.

It worked. Penelope got the part.

You're just starting your second week of our workout program. You may be starting to see some results already, but even if you don't see any changes in your body shape yet, we're sure you are already feeling better about yourself. And that toning of your attitude is just as important as the body shaping we are working on.

When you keep your appointments with yourself, you're keeping your word—you're giving yourself respect. When you see the results—and you will—you'll feel proud of your accomplishments. That's great motivation for any performer.

THIS WEEK'S RUNDOWN

This week we've added repetitions to the exercises we did the first week. You're stronger now and the added reps will challenge your muscles to work harder. The important thing for you now is to stay consistent in your workouts.

As we told you in our chapter on anatomy, muscles gain strength with overload—that is, by being challenged with resistance. That resistance is supplied by weights. The program we have designed for you does not require weights to be effective but if you feel you'd like to challenge your upper body by adding weights and you feel ready to start using weights this week, that's fine.

We suggest that you use weights that will allow you to do the reps in the sets we have designed in good form. So if you find you're having difficulty lifting completely overhead in the Overhead Press, for example, either use lighter weights or go back to using no weights until you're stronger.

If you're just starting to use weights, two- to five-pound hand weights will provide you with the resistance you need to build strength. If you're more advanced, experiment with five to ten pounds. But remember, never sacrifice form for weight.

Week 2

Warm-Up

If you haven't done it yet, before you begin our program this week, try an aerobic activity before you start our exercises. You might want to take a brisk walk, climb stairs in your building or house, or jump rope.

It's most effective if you do at least 20 minutes of aerobic work and then start our exercises. Or if you're pressed for time, you can do 13 minutes of aerobic work and then do our warm-up, which should take you about 7 or 8 minutes.

Just be sure to warm up and stretch your muscles before you start the workout. It's your time to clear your mind and focus on yourself. If you're going to follow our warm-up routine, it's on page 17, and the summary is on page 36.

Once you've completed your warm-up, with your exercise chair nearby, go right into the exercise routine.

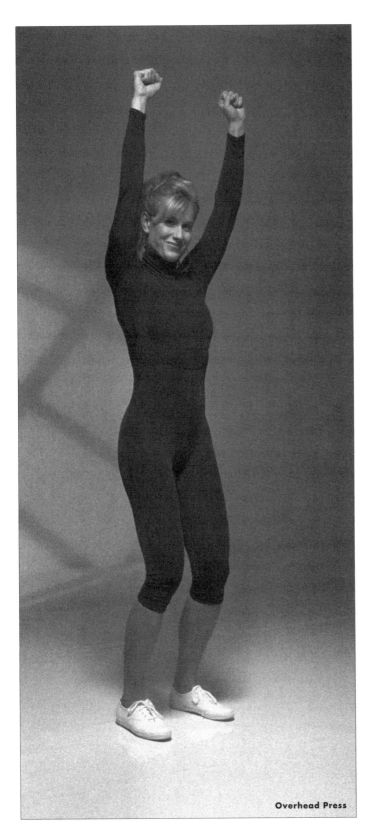

Overhead Press

Overhead Press

Stand in the basic position. (Note: If you feel strong enough, you can work with weights this week. In order to use the weights, just place one in each hand and follow the same directions for form and movement. Remember, you will still get results without weights.) Keep your pelvis neutral while you bend your arms up with your palms forward. Straighten your arms as you lift them until they're fully extended over your head, exhaling as you go. Press up and hold for a beat, then return your arms to their original bent-at-the-elbow position.

Do 12 repetitions to complete 1 set.

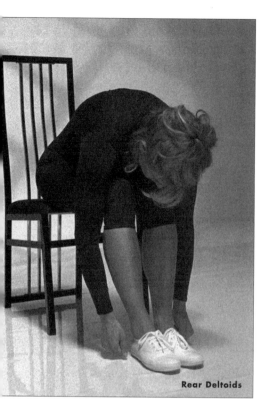

Rear Deltoids

Front Raise

Back to your basic position. Take a deep breath and begin to exhale as you lift your arms, with or without weights, in front of you. Bring them to shoulder height. As you lift, if you are not using actual weights, imagine there are weights sitting on top of your arms and you're lifting them as you raise. Now inhale and lower your arms again. Imagine you're pushing down against the

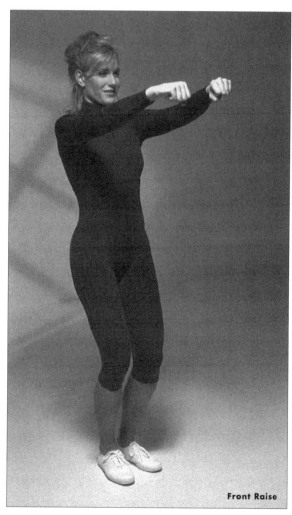

Front Raise

Rear Deltoids

Sit at the edge of your chair and bend forward at the waist. Your arms are down at your sides (with or without hand weights). Now, as you exhale, lift your arms out to the sides and up to shoulder level. Make sure you keep your elbows slightly bent as you squeeze your shoulder blades together. You'll feel the back of your shoulders working. Inhaling, return your arms down so that your fingers are pointed down to the floor.

Remember, don't drop your head. Hold it out as if it were an extension off the top of your spine.

Repeat this move 12 times to complete 1 set.

weights as you lower your arms, palm side down.

Do 12 repetitions to complete 1 set.

Biceps Curls

You're still in your basic standing position. Turn your palms forward and make a loose fist or hold on to your weights. Now curl your arms up toward your shoulders so your fists face your shoulders at the top. Squeeze your biceps as you curl up and when you return your arms to starting position. With or without weights, press down as if there were a heavy weight in your hands giving you resistance. Remember to exhale as you curl up and inhale as you return to starting position.

Even if you're not holding weights in your hands, be careful not to let your wrists move or turn. Keep them steady, with your palms facing up throughout the entire movement.

Do 3 sets of 12 reps.

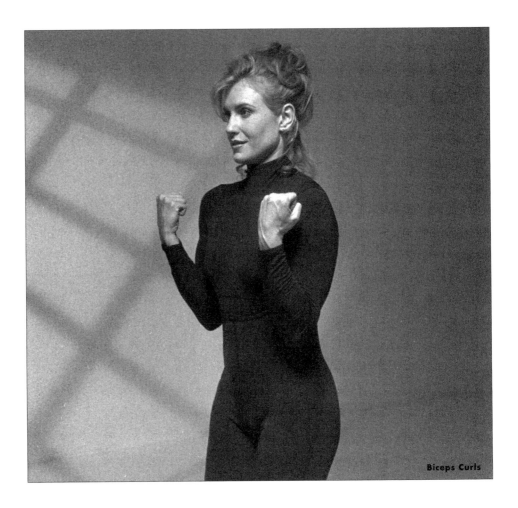

Biceps Curls

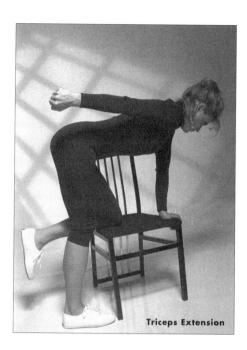

Triceps Extension

Triceps Extension

Let's start with your right arm. Stand on your right leg and place your left knee on your chair. Your torso is extended forward over and parallel to the seat of your chair. Balance your body so your back is flat and steady. Bring your right arm up so your upper arm is parallel to your back. Keep your left knee relaxed to make sure your back is flat.

With your right hand in a loose fist (if you're not holding a weight), palm side facing in toward your body, extend your arm back, keeping the elbow in a straight line with the shoulder. Make sure you exhale and squeeze your triceps on the extension and then inhale as you return down to the starting position.

Do 12 reps of this move and then turn to switch sides.

Rest your right knee on the chair and support your upper body with your right arm. You're standing on your left leg. Bend your upper body from the waist over and parallel to the chair seat. Bend your left arm so that your upper arm is parallel to your back. Your fist (with or without a weight) is facing in toward your body.

Now exhale and extend your left arm back so that it is straight and parallel to the floor. Squeeze the triceps and then inhale, bringing your forearm back down to its original position.

Do 12 reps of this move. By working both arms 12 times each, you have just completed 1 set. Do 2 more sets (a total of 3) of 12 reps on each arm.

You're ready to come back to both feet on the floor and start our lower body work. If you were using weights, set them down but don't put them away.

Pliés

Stand with your legs more than shoulder-width apart. Your toes should be pointed in the 10 and 2 positions of an imaginary clock.

Place your hands on your hips. Lower your body by bending your knees in the direction of your toes. Keep your torso centered and bring your body down so that your butt is almost at a 45-degree angle to your

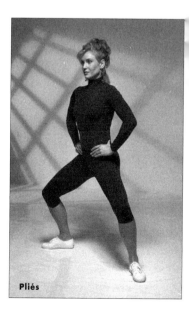

Pliés

knees, and your knees are at a 45-degree angle to your ankles.

Now lift up, squeezing your butt as you lift. Come up to where your knees remain slightly bent. Don't straighten or lock your knees in place.

Do 8 reps of this move to complete 1 set.

Pliés with Pulses

Continue with the plié down but when you get to the bottom, pulse—that is, lift slightly and lower slightly—3 times.

Do 8 reps of this plié pulse to complete 1 set.

Pliés

Return to doing 1 set of 8 reps of the original plié and get ready to work on your:

Hamstrings

Face the back of your chair, resting your forearms on it for support. Make sure you are standing a few

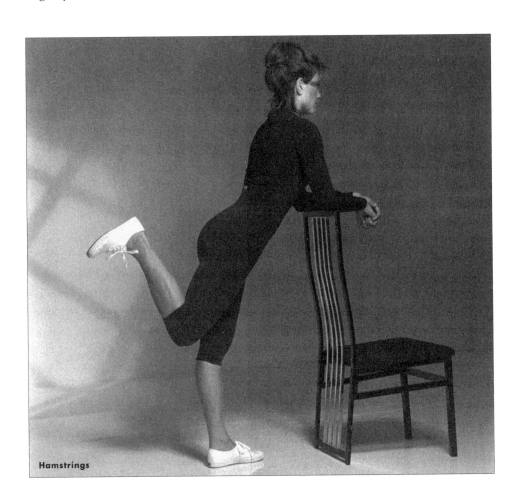

Hamstrings

feet back from the chair. Starting with your left leg straight, but with a relaxed knee, bend your right leg and flex your foot.

Exhale and squeeze your hamstring as you bend the knee. Keep your knees together to help make sure you're isolating your hamstrings. Keep your pelvis in a neutral position as you lift and lower your bent leg.

Do 10 reps with your right leg.

Switch working legs so that you are standing on your right leg. Lift your left leg back, bent at the knee, aiming your left heel back toward your butt, exhaling and squeezing your hamstrings and gluts as you lift. Lower your left leg back to the starting position.

Do 10 reps with the left leg to complete 1 set.

We're moving on to the exercise that was particularly helpful in shaping Penelope Ann's thighs for her role in *Carlito's Way*.

Lunges

Stand with your left side next to the back of the chair. Hold on to the chair for support and bring your right leg forward while your left leg stays back. Raise your left heel and bend your left knee as you lower it toward the floor, going only as low as is comfortable. Do not rest your knee on the floor.

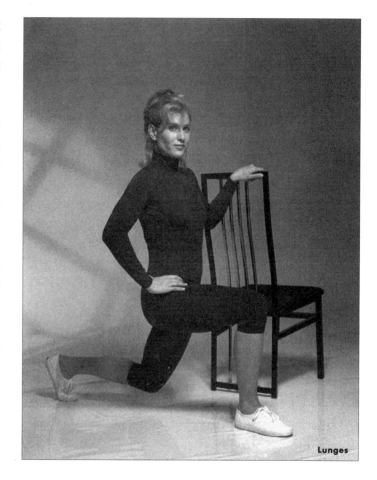

Lunges

Your front (right) leg will, in the lunge position, be at a right angle from your hip to your knee and at a right angle from your knee to your ankle.

Inhale as you move into the lunge position and exhale as you push back off your right leg, using the heel of your right foot to help push you. Squeeze your gluts on the way up.

Repeat the lunge 10 times with your right leg, then switch legs.

Hold on to the chair with your right hand while you extend your left leg forward. Your right leg stays back. Raise your right heel as you bend both legs at the knee. Your front (left) leg bends so that it is at a right angle. The back leg bends so that the knee goes down toward the floor but does not touch the floor.

Hold for a beat and then push up with the weight on your left heel.

Do 10 lunges on your left leg. The 10 lunges on the right leg plus 10 on the left completes 1 set.

Calf Raises

Stand with your feet side-by-side and hold on to your chair for balance. Lift both your heels up, pressing forward onto your toes and then lowering your heels back to the floor.

Do 10 reps of this move.

Calf Raises— Heels Together

Change the position of your feet so that your heels are together and your toes apart. Lift your heels up so that your weight rolls forward onto your toes.

Lift and lower 10 times.

Calf Raises— Toes Together

Change the position of your feet again so that your toes are together and your heels are separated. Once again, roll your weight onto your toes as you lift your heels off the floor. Do 10 reps in this position which works the gastrocnemius. Now let's work the opposite side of the lower leg.

Toe Taps

Standing on both feet, shift your weight onto your right leg and start tapping your left foot. Do this by keeping your heel on the floor, while you raise your left foot as high as you can and then bring it down.

Do 10 taps with your left foot.

Left-to-Right Taps

Here's a new move. Keeping your left heel on the floor, lift your toes and, pivoting on your heel, tap the toes of your left foot out to the left and then arc them over back to the right.

Count each left-to-right move as one. Do 10 Left-to-Right Taps.

Now repeat the set—10 Toe Taps, followed by 10 Left-to-Right Taps—all on the left foot.

Switch feet by shifting your weight onto your left leg and start tapping your right foot, first 10 times up and down and then 10 times arcing right and left.

Repeat the set of 10 Toe Taps plus 10 Right-to-Left Taps—all with your right foot.

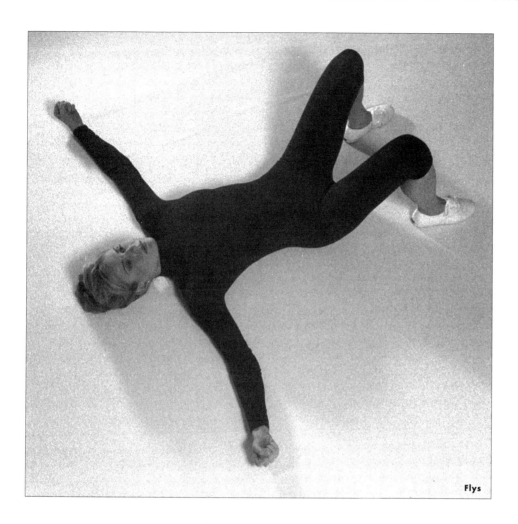

Flys

Calf Stretch

Place your right leg in front of you, bent at the knee. Extend your left leg back comfortably with your heel raised. Now press your left heel down against the floor and hold this stretch for 8 counts.

Switch legs by placing your left leg forward, bent at the knee. Extend your right leg back comfortably with your heel raised. Now press your right heel down against the floor and hold this stretch for 8 counts.

Flys

You can pick up your weights here and get down on the floor, lying on your back with your arms extended up and above your chest. Your legs are bent at the knees with your feet flat on the floor.

Inhale as you slowly lower your arms out to the sides. Keep your elbows slightly bent. Your hands are in a loose fist or holding your weights.

Take your arms back up to their original position as you exhale.

Do 3 sets of 12 reps.

Push-Ups

Begin on your hands and knees. Cross your feet at the ankles. Your hands are parallel with your shoulders. Your fingers are pointing forward and your head is forward with your face looking down toward the floor.

Exhale as you push up, and tighten your abs and squeeze your gluts at the same time. Your back should remain straight. Now inhale and lower again toward the floor but do not rest on the floor; then push up again. When you get to the top, straighten your arms, but do not lock your elbows. Keep them flexible to help you get back down.

Do 8 Push-Ups to complete 1 set, and let's stretch it out with the:

Back Stretch

We borrowed this stretch from yoga. While you're lying on your stomach, lift your right arm and your left leg at the same time. Your lifted foot should be flexed with your toes pointing down. As you stretch your arm and your leg as far as you can, exhale, then breathe deeply as you hold the stretch for a count of 8.

Switch so that your left arm and right leg are lifted and stretching. Exhale on the lift and breathe deeply for a count of 8. Now get back up on your hands and knees.

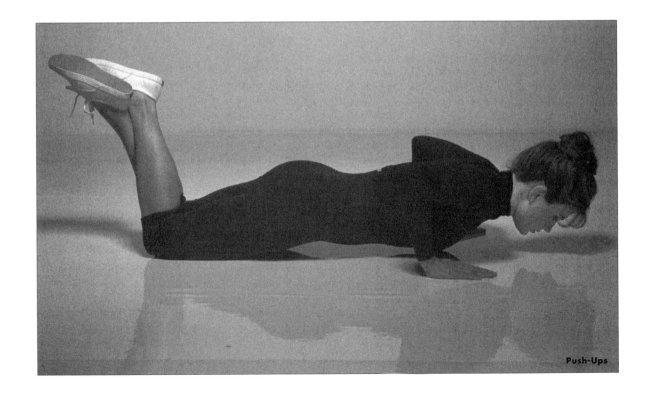

Push-Ups

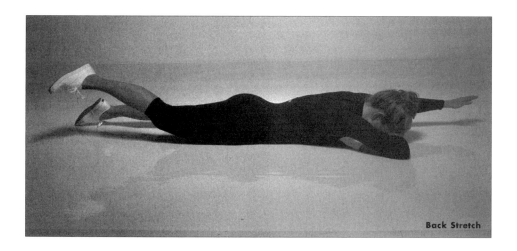

Back Stretch

Bent Leg Raise

We're fighting gravity on this one—both literally and figuratively. This exercise will help your butt and firm up the hamstrings (the back of the thigh).

Make sure your knees are positioned right below your hips, and your elbows are positioned below your shoulders with your hands out in front of you. Keep your back straight—don't sink in the middle—and pull in your abs as if they're going up against your spine.

Now raise your right leg, with your knee bent and your right foot flexed. Exhale on the lift, pulling in on your abs. Get your knee up and level with your butt and squeeze your hamstring and glut. Now inhale as you lower your still-bent leg back down to the starting position. Then squeeze up again.

Do 1 set of 10 reps with your right leg.

Now lift your left leg so that your left quad is facing the floor and the sole of your left foot is facing the ceiling. Exhale on the lift and inhale when you bring your left leg back down to its original position. Do 1 set of 10 reps with your left leg.

Let's get ready to work the outer and inner thighs starting with abduction.

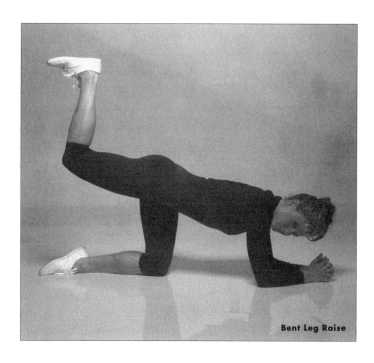

Bent Leg Raise

Side Leg Lift

Lie down on your left side so that your right hip is over your left hip. Your knees are bent at an angle so that they slant out from your hips. Your bottom arm is bent at the elbow and your head is resting on your left hand. Your right arm is out in front of your chest, acting as an anchor.

Now exhale as you lift your top leg. Be careful not to lift only your knee or to lead with your knee. Lift your entire right leg as far as you can without rolling back. Then bring your right leg down, squeezing your butt together, but do not rest or touch your bottom leg before you lift your right leg up again.

Do 3 sets of 10 reps and switch legs.

Now lying on your right side with your legs together and extended forward with your knees bent, lift your left leg up. Inhale as you lower your leg and squeeze your butt, then repeat the move.

Do 3 sets of 10 reps and then go back to your left side to work the adductors with the:

Bottom Leg Lift

Your body is lying in a straight line, with your head resting on your outstretched lower arm. Place your upper arm in front of you for support. Bring your top leg over in front of you, keeping your knee lifted. Flex your bottom foot.

Now, without moving the rest of your body, lift your lower leg. Lower the left leg but do not let it touch the floor before you lift it again.

Do 3 sets of 10 lifts.

Turn to the other side and start working your right inner thigh.

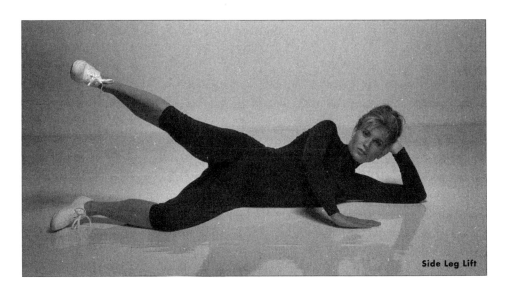

Side Leg Lift

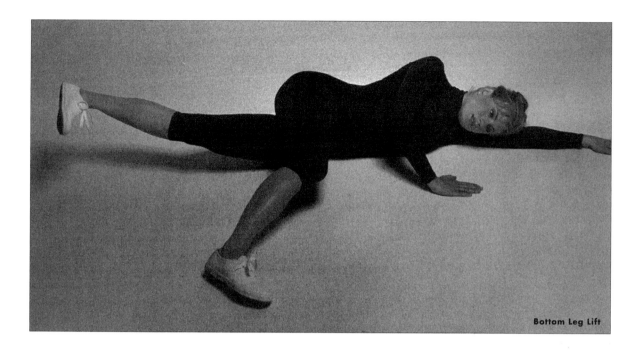

Bottom Leg Lift

Lying on your right side with your legs together, extend the upper leg out in front of you and rest your head on your right hand. Exhale and lift up your right leg so that the inside of your thigh is squeezing up toward the ceiling. Lower that leg but don't rest it—lift it again.

Do 3 sets of 10 lifts.

Abdominals

Crunches

Lie on the floor on your back. Bring your knees up with your feet flat on the floor in front of you. With your hands behind your head and your chin up off your chest, lift your shoulders off the floor and up toward your knees. Exhale on the lift up and inhale as you go back down. Do not rest your upper back on the floor when you come down; exhale and lift again.

Do 10 reps to complete 1 set.

Crunches with Pulses

Rest a beat, then repeat the same move but this time pulse 3 times when you get to the top of your lift. Make sure that your abs are pulled in when you pulse and that you inhale as you go back down. Do not let your upper back touch the floor.

Do 10 reps of the pulse lift to complete 1 set.

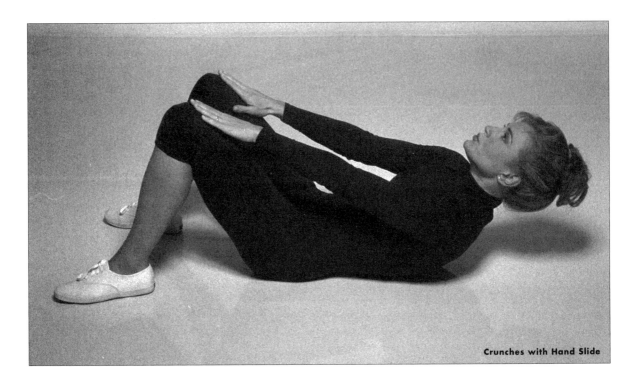

Crunches with Hand Slide

Crunches with Hand Slide

Take your hands out from behind your neck and place them on your quads. Lift your upper body using your abs while you exhale and slide your hands up your quads toward your knees. Inhale as you return down but don't take your hands off your quads.

Do 10 of these slide lifts to complete 1 set.

Elbow-to-Knee Crunches

Take your hands off your quads and put them behind your head, resting your head in your hands. Your elbows are pointed outward. Now bring your left leg up so that your left ankle is resting on your right knee. Exhale as you lift, pulling in on your abs, and point your right elbow up and over your left knee. Do not twist your spine. Inhale as you lower.

Do a total of 10 reps to complete 1 set.

Now switch sides. Place your right ankle on your left knee. Lift your shoulders and point your left elbow up and over your right knee. Exhale on the lift and inhale as you go back down.

Do 10 reps to complete 1 set.

Crunches

Bring your shoulders down to the floor and then bring your right leg down so both your feet are resting on the floor. You're back in your original crunch position.

With your hands still behind your head, lift your shoulders up off the floor, pulling in on your abs as you exhale. Do not use your hands to pull up your head—use your abs to pull you up. Then inhale as you go back down but don't rest on the floor; lift again.

Do 10 reps to complete your abs workout.

Cool-Down

Lie back and rest for a moment before you start your cool-down stretches, which begin on page 49.

Do this workout four times this week. And have a good time doing it. Remember, you're working toward a goal; and when you see the approval in your fans' eyes, it will all be worth it.

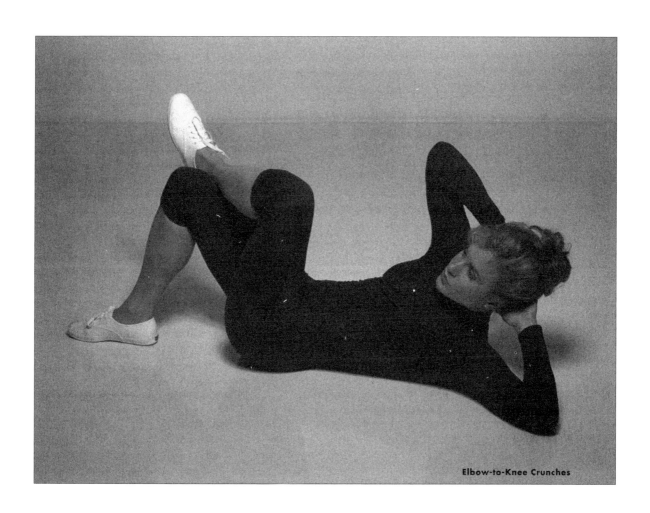

Elbow-to-Knee Crunches

WEEK 2 SUMMARY

Exercise	Reps	Sets
Overhead Press	12	1
Rear Deltoids	12	1
Front Raise	12	1
Biceps Curls	12	3
Triceps Extension	12 right/12 left	3
Pliés	8	1
Pliés with Pulses	8	1
Pliés	8	1
Hamstrings	10 right/10 left	1
Lunges	10 right/10 left	1
Calf Raises	10	1
Calf Raises—Heels Together	10	1
Calf Raises—Toes Together	10	1
Toe Taps	10 right/10 left	2
Left-to-Right (and Right-to-Left) Taps	10 left/10 right	2
Calf Stretch	hold 8 counts each side	
Flys	12	3
Push-Ups	8	1
Back Stretch	hold 8 counts each side	
Bent Leg Raise	10 right/10 left	1
Side Leg Lift	10 right/10 left	3
Bottom Leg Lift	10 right/10 left	3
Crunches	10	1
Crunches with Pulses	10	1
Crunches with Hand Slide	10	1
Elbow-to-Knee Crunches	10 right/10 left	1
Crunches	10	1

6

Directing Your Action

Week 3: Repetition Is the Key Requirement

By now, you have most likely decided which exercise you like the best and which you like the least (the least favorite is usually the one that's the hardest to do). No matter which move is your favorite, we hope you're getting into a new habit—the workout habit.

If you're having a tough time convincing yourself that you truly enjoy working out, don't feel discouraged; don't even feel bad. You're in good company. For most people, working up to working out is a difficult task, and a lot of people will tell you that working out is a lot more fun after it's finished.

When we asked Michelle Pfeiffer what she likes least about working out she answered, "Working out." And when we asked what she likes best about working out, she answered, "How I feel afterward."

Pam Dawber doesn't like to work out alone, so she gets a friend or friends together for her workout sessions.

When it comes to doing push-ups, Candice Bergen always says, "I can't do that." Then she does 'that' and says, " 'that' felt great."

We tell you these things because we know that sometimes no matter how motivated you are to get results, you still may be inclined to give up. Intimidation, negativity, or shortsightedness can make it hard to get past the workout—from imagining the results to actually seeing the results.

Actors are trained to be in touch with their emotions. They work constantly at ridding themselves of personal obstacles that keep them from getting at the characters they're playing. They work with the directors of their projects to explore circumstances, patterns of behavior, and even movement that is true to their character.

Actors can apply this training to situations in their own lives. Michelle, Candice, and Pam, for example, are able to figure out how to get past any blocks that they have against exercise.

You can direct yourself to achieve the same kinds of results. Explore the environment in which you work best. Discover the circumstances that encourage you to work out most regularly. Then create those circumstances and that environment. Be honest about which exercise you find the most challenging and make up your mind that, if you really focus on it, you're going to make it work for you.

Whenever we do lunges, Michelle gives the "this is too hard—do we have to?" look, but she does them all anyway. The next day Michelle will open the door and say how great she feels—the lunges made her feel tight, toned, and a little sore, too.

So if you run into difficulty with any of the exercises, don't skip them or attach negative feelings to them. Instead, think of the positive results you're going to get and get going!

This Week's Plan

We're adding on again this week. We've got more repetitions of the familiar exercises and we've added some new moves. Your muscles have been building up their endurance and it will take more reps to challenge them. Next week we're going to further challenge your muscles by adding supersets* to your workout. So this week is very important in building up to that next stage. If you haven't started using weights yet, this would be a good week to pick them up.

Week 3

Warm-Up

You can start by doing your own aerobic warm-up along with the primetime warm-up or you can start with just our warm-up. Remember, you should warm up before you start the actual program. The warm-up will help you reduce the risk of in-

*A superset puts 2 or more exercises together that work opposing muscle groups without a break between sets.

juries and will give you a chance to focus your mind's eye on you.

Turn back to page 17 for our warm-up.

After you've completed the warm-up, go right into your exercise routine:

Overhead Press

Stand in your basic position with your arms down at your sides. Moving only your arms, bend them up with your palms facing forward, then straighten them as you lift overhead. Your end point is above your head with your arms fully extended. Exhale as you move your arms up and hold them for a beat at the top. Now return your arms to their original position, which is bent at the elbow.

If you are using weights, hold 1 in each hand and follow the same instructions.

Do 15 repetitions to complete 1 set.

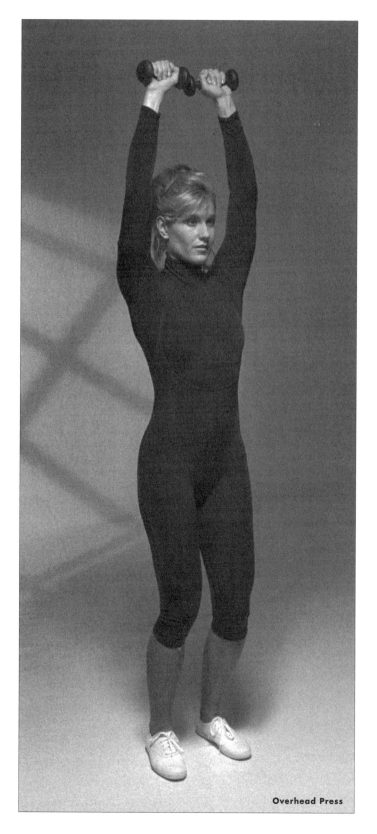

Overhead Press

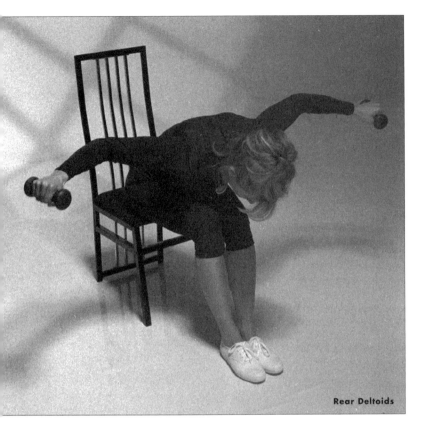

Rear Deltoids

Front Raise

Standing in the basic position again, exhale as you lift your arms in front of you, bringing them (with or without weights) up to shoulder height. Don't lift them quickly—make sure you feel the lift against gravity as you raise your arms. Inhale as you slowly lower your arms, working your arms against the resistance of

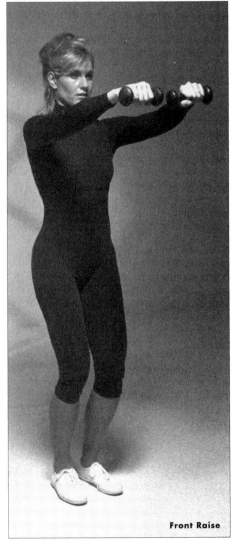

Front Raise

Rear Deltoids

Sit on the edge of your chair with your arms down at your sides and bend forward at the waist. Exhale as you lift your arms (with or without weights) out to the side and up to shoulder level. Squeeze your shoulder blades together, keeping your elbows slightly bent. Your head stays level with your spine. Then on the inhale, return your arms down to your sides, palm side toward the floor. If you are holding weights, grasp them lightly. Be careful not to move your wrists around. Keep them steady.

Do 15 reps to complete 1 set.

imaginary weights or controlling the pull of the real weights.

Do 15 reps to complete 1 set.

Biceps Curls— Angled

These biceps curls are a little different from what we've been doing. By changing the angle of the lift, you'll gain more strength all around your arm.

Start with your arms down at your sides and your hands held in a loose fist or holding your weights, palms facing outward but angled slightly inward. This time, when you bend your elbows and curl up your arms, curl them at a 45-degree angle so that your palms are facing each other instead of facing your chest. You'll feel your biceps working; you'll feel it in your shoulders too.

Do 3 sets of 15 reps.

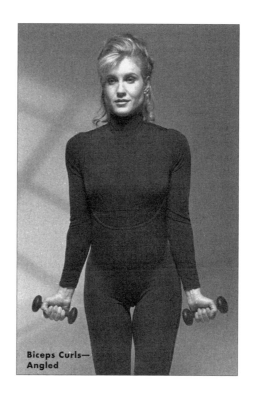

Biceps Curls— Angled

Triceps Dips

We've got a new and more intense triceps exercise this week.

Stand with your back toward the seat of your chair. Place your hands behind you on the chair seat. (You'll have to bring your knees out in front of you and lower yourself to the chair seat's height.) With your elbows slightly bent and your fingers facing forward, start with your butt and

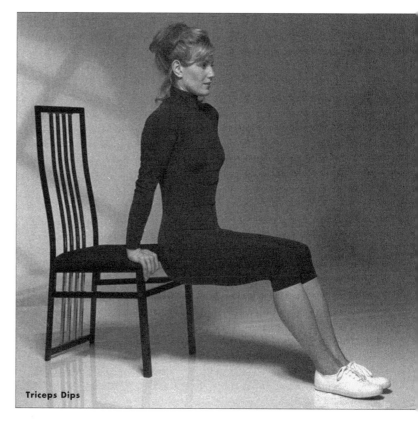

Triceps Dips

thighs at chair-seat level and dip down so that your butt and your back skim the chair as you lower. Go down only as far as is comfortable.*

As you get stronger it will get easier for you to go lower, but don't touch the floor with your butt. Inhale as you dip down and exhale as you lift up.

Do 2 sets of 10 reps each.

Pliés

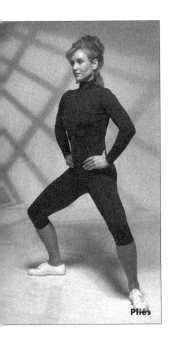

Pliés

Step onto the face of that imaginary clock so that your feet land on the 10 and 2 positions. Place your legs more than shoulder-width apart and rest your hands on your hips.

Tighten both sides of your butt and lower your body as you bend your knees, which should point out over your toes. Do not move your torso—keep it steady as you move lower. Bring your butt down so it's almost as low as your knees. Your knees should be at a 45-degree angle to your ankles.

Now lift, squeezing your butt as you go. Stop while your knees are still slightly bent, keeping the tension on the inner thighs. Do 8 reps to complete 1 set.

Note: If your chair is too high for you at the beginning, start doing the Triceps Dips on a step in your house or by using a low sofa until you feel comfortable dipping from chair height.

Pliés with Pulses

Continue with the regular plié down, but at the bottom; pulse 3 times. The pulse is a slight move up and down to add intensity to the work. Keep your butt tight.

Do 8 reps to complete 1 set.

Pliés

Now do 8 reps of the regular plié to complete 1 set.

Now go back to your chair. You've just worked the inner thigh and gluts and you're about to work the hamstrings and gluts.

Hamstrings

Standing a few feet away, face the back of the chair and rest your forearms on it for support. Shift your weight onto your left leg, which is straight but with a relaxed knee. Now lift up your right leg and bend it back at the knee. Flex your foot. Keep your knees close together.

Exhale and squeeze your gluts and hamstrings as you raise your foot, aiming your heel toward your butt. Then lower your foot down to starting position.

Do 10 reps to complete 1 set. Now switch working legs.

Stand on your right leg, which is straight but with a relaxed knee. Lift your left leg up behind you and

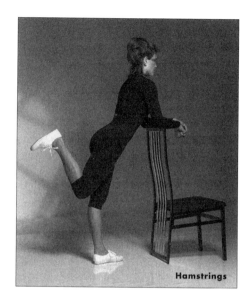

Hamstrings

bend it back at the knee. Lift and lower your upper leg as you squeeze your gluts and your hamstrings. Exhale on the lift and inhale on the lower.

Do 10 reps to complete 1 set. We're moving on to a new way of doing lunges:

Four-Count Lunges

You can do four-count lunges without the chair, but if you still feel a bit shaky, hold on to the chair for support. If you don't use the chair, you can hold your arms out to the side for balance.

The counts are: (1) step, (2) press down, (3) push up, and (4) step back.

Let's start with the right leg lunge. Keep your left leg back as you take a big step forward with your right leg and lower down so

that your butt is at knee level. Your left heel will come up as you lower. Then push up with your weight on your right heel and step back to your original position.

Do 10 reps on your right leg to complete 1 set. Then switch legs.

Your right leg is now the back leg. Step forward with your left leg and lower your butt down to knee level. Your right heel will come up as you lower. Now push up with your weight on your left heel and step back with your left leg.

Do 10 reps on your left leg to complete 1 set.

Lunges are the exercise that Michelle Pfeiffer loves to hate. Here's one you won't hate, but you sure will feel it!

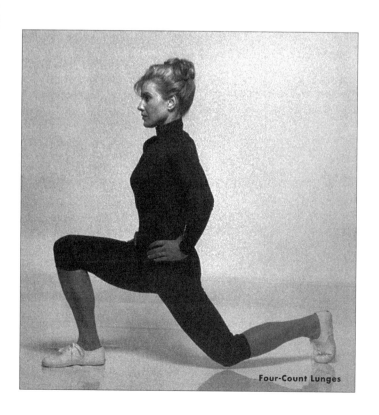

Four-Count Lunges

Calf Raises

Stand behind the chair and hold on to it for balance, with your legs very slightly apart and your feet facing forward.

Now lift both heels up, pressing forward onto your toes, and then lower your heels back to the floor. Keep breathing—exhale as you lift and inhale as you lower. Remember to keep working your abs by inhaling and exhaling.

Do 10 reps to complete 1 set.

Calf Raises— Heels Together

Change the position of your feet so that your heels are together and your toes are apart. Now lift and lower 10 times to complete 1 set.

Calf Raises— Toes Together

Change your position so that your toes are together and your heels are apart. Lift and lower 10 times to complete 1 set. Now that we've worked the gastrocnemius, let's work the front of the lower leg.

Toe Taps

Standing straight, shift your weight onto your right leg and start tap-ping your left foot. Tap by raising your toes up while your heel remains on the floor. Bring your toes up as far as you can so you can feel the flex at the front of your ankle.

Do 10 taps with your left foot.

Left-to-Right Taps

Now do the side-to-side tap with your left heel on the floor and lifting your toes, pointing them first to the right and then to the left.

Each right-to-left move is 1 rep. Do 10 reps with your left foot.

Now repeat the set—10 Toe Taps and 10 Right-to-Left Taps—still with your left foot.

Now switch feet. Shift your weight onto your left leg and start tapping your right foot. Do 10 Toe Taps and then do 10 Left-to-Right Taps to complete the set.

Then repeat the set with the same foot. This next stretch will feel pretty good right now.

Calf Stretch

Place your right leg in front of you and bend it at the knee. Extend your left leg behind you with your heel raised. Now press your left heel down against the floor, stretching the soleus. Hold this stretch for 8 counts.

Switch working legs. Place your left leg forward, bent at the knee. Extend your right leg backward with your heel raised. Now press your right heel against the floor and hold this stretch for 8 counts.

Now it's time for our floor work.

Flys

Lie on your back with your arms extended up over your chest. Bring your knees up and keep your feet flat on the floor. Make loose fists with your hands or hold on to your weights. Inhale as you slowly lower your arms down to the floor. Exhale as you return your arms back up to their original position.

Do 3 sets of 15 reps. Prepare for Push-Ups.

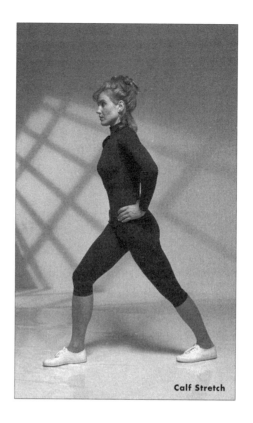

Calf Stretch

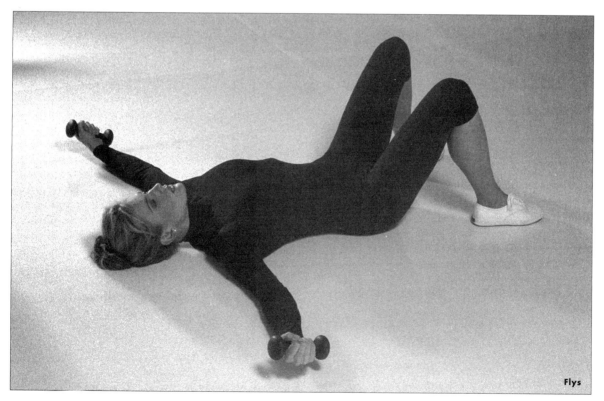

Flys

Push-Ups

Begin on your hands and knees, with your feet up, soles facing the ceiling and crossed at the ankles. Place your hands on the floor, lined up under your shoulders. Point your fingers forward.

Inhale as you lower your upper body, skimming the floor but not resting on it. Then exhale as you push up with your arms. Tighten your abs and your butt as you lift, and be care-ful not to arch your back or let it sink in the middle. Your back should be straight, and your head should be forward.

Do 10 reps to complete 1 set. Stay in the pushed-up position.

Bent Leg Raise— Extend

This week there's a new twist to this exercise. Lower your upper body to rest on your elbows. Push back so that you're resting on your bent knees and your weight is evenly distributed over your torso. Pull in on your abs and raise your right leg, keeping your knee bent and the sole of your foot pointing toward the ceiling. Raise it until you can feel the tightening of the hamstring and gluts. Now extend your leg so it's straight out and then bring your heel in toward your butt, squeezing your gluts. Extend it back out, keeping your knee bent, and lift. Then bring it back in.

Do 10 reps and switch legs.

Still on your elbows and knees, raise your left leg and bend it at the knee. Squeeze your gluts as you lift your foot toward the ceiling, and then extend it straight out. Squeeze your hamstrings and butt as you bring your left heel toward your butt.

Do 10 reps and come down off your elbows and knees and onto your stomach.

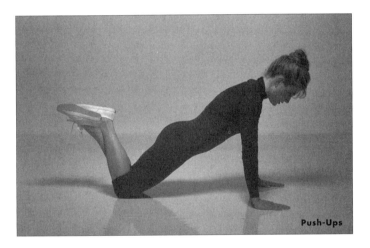

Push-Ups

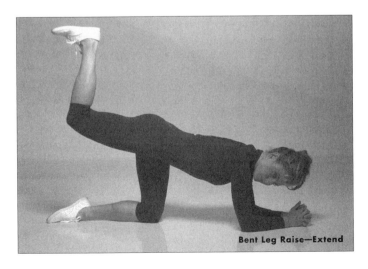

Bent Leg Raise—Extend

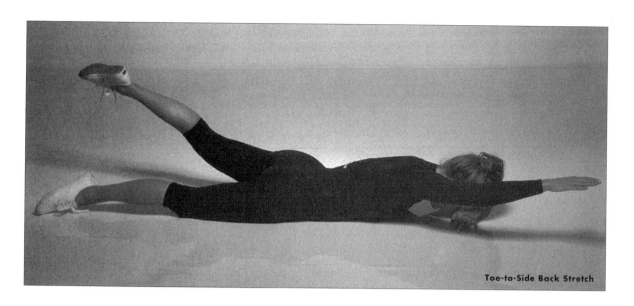

Toe-to-Side Back Stretch

Toe-to-Side Back Stretch

This week, instead of keeping your toes pointed to the floor, you'll be turning the toes of each foot out to the side. Start by lying on the floor with your arms and legs stretched out straight. Now lift your right arm and left leg off the floor. Turn your left foot out to the side so that your toes are pointing left. Hold for a count of 8 and then return to your original position.

Switch so that your left arm and right leg lift together. Turn your right foot out to the side, toes pointing right, as you lift and hold for 8 counts.

By turning your toes out to the side you work more of the side of the glut along with the back of the glut. Now get ready to work the sides of your thighs.

Side Leg Lift

Start by lying on your left side, hips stacked straight (not leaning forward or backward), knees bent out between 45 degrees and 90 degrees from your upper body. Your legs should mirror each other—the inside of the top knee should look down on the inside of the lower knee. Flex your right foot.

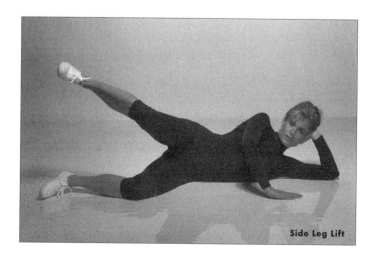

Side Leg Lift

Bend your left arm at the elbow and rest your head in your hand. Place your right arm in front of you as an anchor, to keep you from rocking back when you lift your right leg. Lift up, working against gravity. You'll feel the tension in the outer thigh and the side of your butt.

As you bring down the right leg, squeeze your gluts together and squeeze your inner thigh muscles, but don't bring your legs completely together. Imagine you have a big ball resting on your bottom leg.

Do 3 sets of 12 reps. Switch sides.

Turn over so you are lying on your right side, with your hips straight and your legs together. Flex your left foot and place your left arm in front of you to hold your upper body in a steady position. Rest your head on your right hand.

Now, without tipping back or rolling forward, lift your left leg up, pushing against gravity. Then lower it as if you were squeezing that imaginary ball. Keep your gluts squeezed throughout.

Do 3 sets of 12 reps. Move on to work your adductors.

Bottom Leg Lift

Go back to lying on your left side with your left arm, your torso, and your left leg in a straight line. Bring your right leg and arm in front of you with your knee bent slightly.

Lift and lower your bottom leg with your foot flexed. Do not touch the floor when you lower your leg.

Do 3 sets of 12 reps, with the following variations:

When you lift your leg in the second set, point your foot.

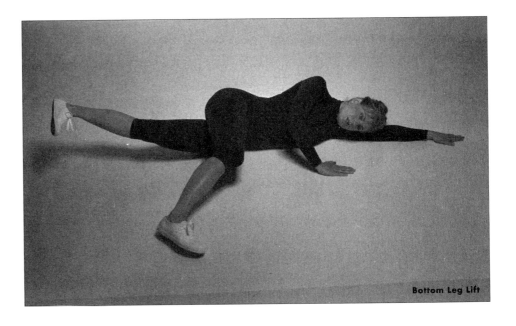

Bottom Leg Lift

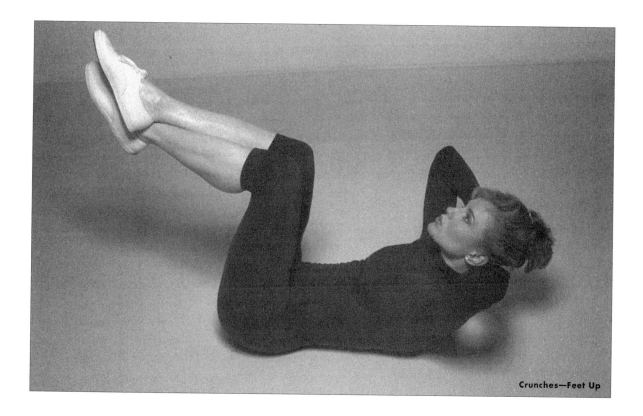

Crunches—Feet Up

But when you lift your leg in the third set, flex your foot on the way up and point it on the way down.

Switch sides so that your right leg is on the bottom, in a straight line with your torso and right arm. Rest your head on your right arm and extend your left arm in front of you. Place your left leg forward, bent at the knee.

Lift and lower your bottom leg, squeezing your inner thigh muscles and flexing your right foot. When you lower your leg do not touch the floor.

Do 3 sets of 12 reps.

When you lift your leg in the second set, point your foot.

When you lift your leg in the third set, flex your foot on the way up and point it on the way down.

Abdominals

We're adding on to the reps you did the first two weeks and giving you different moves, so follow the rundown carefully.

Crunches—Feet Up

Start on your back with your knees and feet raised up in the air over your hips. Cross your ankles and place your hands behind your head with your head resting in your hands.

Now lift your shoulders up off the floor—remember not to pull on your head or neck—using your abs to bring your upper body up toward your bent knees. Keep your knees steady. Exhale as you come up and inhale as you go back down. Remember not to let your shoulders or upper back touch the floor.

Do 10 reps to complete 1 set.

Crunches with Pulses

Now lift again, but this time when you get your upper body lifted toward your knees, pulse 3 times before you lower.

Do 10 reps to complete 1 set.

Two-Count Crunches

For this set you're going to lift up in 2 counts. So you lift halfway on count 1, then lift again as high as you can on count 2. Now lower halfway for the first count and then down to your original position for the second count. Remember to exhale when you lift, so you feel those abs contracting, and inhale as you go down the 2 counts.

Now do 10 reps to complete 1 set.

Crunches with Pulses

Next, repeat the pulse move. That is, lift your shoulders up toward your knees and pulse 3 times at the top.

Do 10 reps to complete 1 set.

Crunches

Now do the original crunches by lifting your upper body in one move toward your knees and then lowering again.

Do 10 reps to complete 1 set.

Crunches—Feet Up— Elbow to Knee

Now we're going to help shape your waist by working your obliques, which are at your sides.

Lift your knees and feet up in the air and place your hands behind your head. Lift so that your left shoulder and elbow aim toward your right knee. Do not bring your elbow in and do not twist your spine.

Do 5 reps with the left elbow.

Then alternate sides, remembering to exhale on the lift as you aim your right shoulder and elbow toward your left knee. Inhale down.

Do 5 reps with your right elbow.

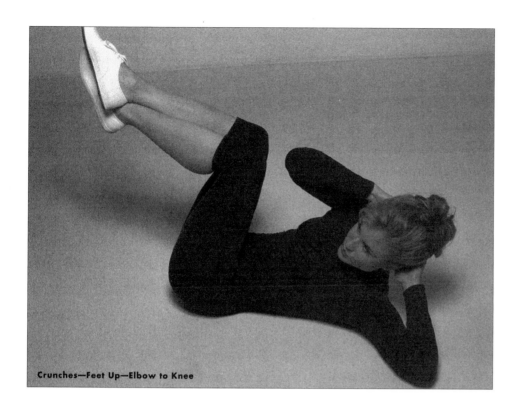

Crunches—Feet Up—Elbow to Knee

Crunches—Feet Up—Alternating Elbow to Knee

Now do the same move, except you'll alternate right and left sides. Start by lifting your left elbow and shoulder toward your right knee and lower. Then lift your right elbow and shoulder toward your left knee and lower. Do 10 reps alternating left and right to complete 1 set.

Crunches with Pulses

Return to the 3 pulses at the top.
    Do 10 reps to complete 1 set.

Crunches

Do the original crunches by lifting your upper body toward your knees and coming right back down.
    Do 10 reps to complete your last set.

Cool-Down

Now lie back and breathe deeply. You're done with the abs work. And after you finish your cool-down, you'll be halfway through our program. You're doing great! But don't stop now. Cool down first with the cool-down stretches on page 49.

WEEK 3 SUMMARY

Exercise	Reps	Set
Overhead Press	15	1
Rear Deltoids	15	1
Front Raise	15	1
Biceps Curls—Angled	15	3
Triceps Dips	10	2
Pliés	8	1
Pliés with Pulses	8	1
Pliés	8	1
Hamstrings	10 right/10 left	1
Four-Count Lunges	10 right/10 left	1
Calf Raises	10	1
Calf Raises—Heels Together	10	1
Calf Raises—Toes Together	10	1
Toe Taps	10 right/10 left	2
Left-to-Right (and Right-to-Left) Taps	10 left/10 right	2
Calf Stretch	hold 8 counts each side	
Flys	15	3
Push-Ups	10	1
Bent Leg Raise—Extend	10 right/10 left	1
Toe-to-Side Back Stretch	hold 8 counts each side	
Side Leg Lift	12 right/12 left	3
Bottom Leg Lift	12 right/12 left	3
Crunches—Feet Up	10	1
Crunches with Pulses	10	1
Two-Count Crunches	10	1
Crunches with Pulses	10	1
Crunches	10	1
Crunches—Feet Up—Elbow to Knee	5 left/5 right	1
Crunches—Feet Up—Alternating Elbow to Knee	10	1
Crunches with Pulses	10	1
Crunches	10	1

7

Adding a New Twist to the Plot

Week 4: New Moves Keep the Action Exciting

By now, your fourth week into the program, you've pretty much got the routine down—so it's time to change it. It's just like a movie. As soon as you get to know the characters and their needs, things change so the action stays exciting and you stay interested.

We want you to stay interested and challenged with our primetime program. Think about the stage actress who successfully plays the same role over and over—maybe hundreds of times. She finds ways to bring life into each and every performance, by challenging herself to fine-tune each and every line and movement. It's not much different from what you have to do. Exercise is a repeat performance—you constantly have to fine-tune every move. But unlike a stage script, our script is dynamic—more like episodic television. Same characters, same set, but a different story every week. Our story this week adds supersets.

Supersets are groups of two or more exercises that work opposing muscle groups without a break between sets. Muscles are challenged through repetition, and supersets give you the chance to do more moves in less time.

Successful exercise requires complete focus and attention. If you're easily distracted, you've got to find a way to make sure you don't give in to those distractions.

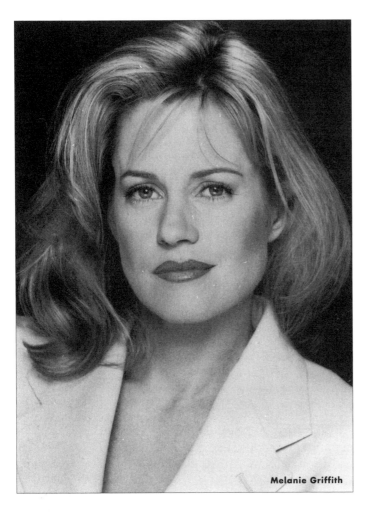

Melanie Griffith

That's what we did with Melanie Griffith. When we worked out at her home, the kids and the ever-ringing phone were always requiring her attention. We didn't get a lot of reps in before we were interrupted. So we did shorter sets and super-sets in order to get results. We also began hiking outside. That way we were able to concentrate strictly on exercise. We want you to do the same—don't let outside distractions break up your act. Your show must go on if you want to join other primetime bodies.

Week 4

Warm-Up

Start with your own 20-minute aer-obic workout, or do a combination of 13 minutes of aerobics and our 7-minute warm-up routine. The prime-time warm-up begins on page 17.

After you've completed your warm-up session, get ready for the new moves we have for you this week. We'll start with our first su-perset. The exercises are familiar in form but they're more intense.

If you haven't used weights yet, and you feel strong enough, you could start using weights this week. If you have already used weights, you might want to try using heavier weights this week, even though the supersetting alone gives you an added challenge. If at any time, the weights feel too heavy, put them down and work with no weights. And if you choose to work without weights, follow the instructions as given, since the moves are the same with or without weights.

SUPERSET:
Overhead Press and Biceps Curls

Overhead Press

Get into your basic standing position with your legs shoulder-width apart and your knees bent slightly. Your arms, holding weights, are down at your sides.

Standing steady, bring up your arms, bending them with your palms facing forward. Now straighten them as you lift overhead. Bring them up so that your arms are fully extended overhead; hold for a beat and lower your arms to their bent-at-the-elbow starting position. Remember to exhale on the lift and inhale when you bring your arms down.

Do 10 reps to complete 1 set and immediately start your Biceps Curls.

Biceps Curls—Angled

Bring your arms back down to your sides, still holding your weights. Your palms should face outward and be angled slightly inward. Now bend your elbows and curl up your arms, bringing them up at a 45-degree angle so that your palms and weights wind up facing each other on opposite sides of your chest.

Do 10 reps to complete 1 set.

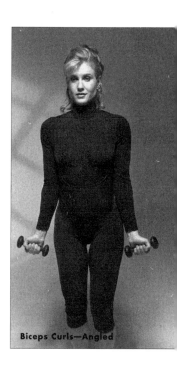

Biceps Curls—Angled

Overhead Press/Biceps Curls

Repeat both the Overhead Press (1 set of 10 reps) and the Biceps Curls (1 set of 10 reps).

You have now completed your first superset. Let's move on to your next superset.

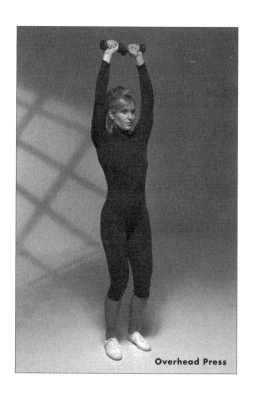

Overhead Press

SUPERSET:
Triceps Extension and Rear Deltoids

Triceps Extension— Palm Up

Go to your chair and place your left knee on the seat of the chair. Stand on your right leg and extend your torso forward so that your chest is parallel to the chair seat. Your back is flat and your body is steady. Hold a weight in your right hand and bring your right arm up so your upper arm is parallel to your back.

Now with your right hand facing in toward your body, extend your arm back, keeping the elbow in a

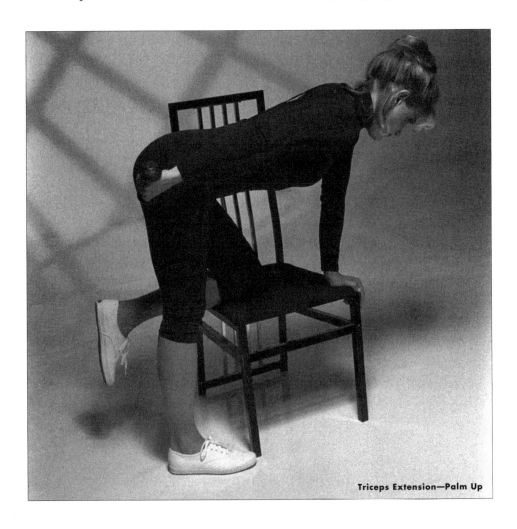

Triceps Extension—Palm Up

straight line with your shoulder. Exhale on the extension as you squeeze your triceps, turning your palm up to the ceiling. Now return to the starting position.

Do 10 reps on the right arm to complete 1 set. Then sit down on the edge of your chair to start right into your first Rear Deltoids set.

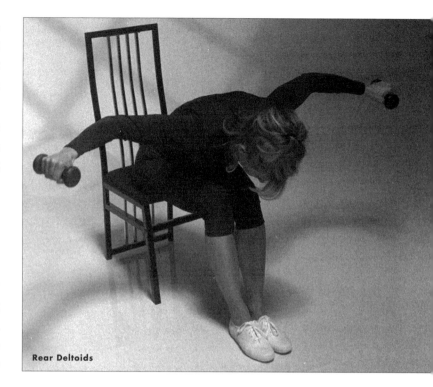

Rear Deltoids

Rear Deltoids

Bend forward at the waist with your arms at your sides. You're holding weights in both your hands. As you exhale, lift your arms out to the sides and bring them up to shoulder level. Squeeze your shoulder blades together, then inhale and release your arms back down so that your knuckles are facing the floor. Be sure to hold your head out as if it were an extension of your spine.

Do 10 reps to complete 1 set. Put down one of your weights and get ready to repeat the Triceps Extension.

Triceps Extension— Palm Up

We'll work your left arm this time. Place your right knee on the chair and keep your left leg on the floor. Bend your upper body over so that it is parallel to the chair seat. Bring your left arm up so that your upper

arm is parallel to your back. Your left elbow should be bent and level with your shoulder. Your fist is facing in toward your body.

Now extend your left arm back so that it is straight, and as you squeeze your triceps, turn your palm up to the ceiling. Bring your arm down.

Do 10 reps on the left arm to complete 1 set.

Rear Deltoids

Get back on the edge of the chair with weights in both hands and finish with another set of 10 Rear Deltoids repetitions. Get ready for your third upper body superset.

SUPERSET:
Front Raise and Triceps Dips

Front Raise

Stand in the basic position with your knees slightly bent and your weights in both hands. Exhale as you lift both your arms up in front of you, bringing them up to shoulder height, palms facing down. Then inhale as you slowly lower your arms.

Do 10 reps to complete 1 set. Put down your weights and go directly back to the chair.

Triceps Dips

Sit on the edge of your chair with your hands on the front edge of the

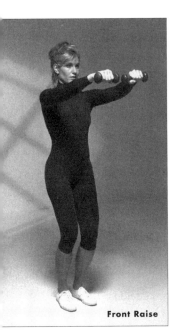

Front Raise

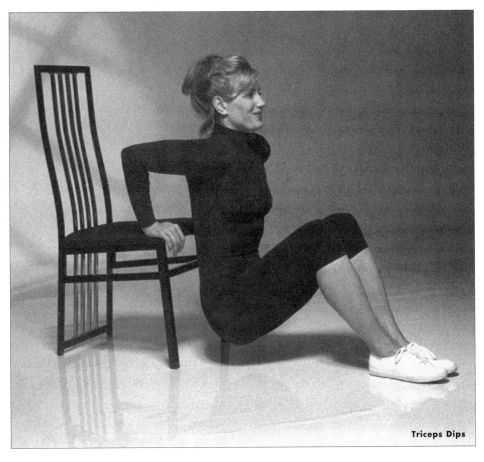

Triceps Dips

seat and your legs out in front of you, knees bent. Start with your butt at chair level and dip down so that your butt and your back skim the chair as you lower. Don't touch the floor with your butt. Now exhale and lift back up.

Do 10 reps to complete 1 set.

Front Raises/ Triceps Dips

Stand up and lift your weights for the second set of 10 Front Raises. Remember to keep your wrists steady and to breathe—always exhaling on the exertion (lift).

Now without delay, do another set of 10 Triceps Dips—then put down your weights. We're moving on to work your inner thighs and gluts with our:

Two-Count Pliés

We have a new plié move for you this week. First, get into position: your feet on the 10 and 2 positions of a clock, slightly more than shoulder-width apart, and your knees slightly bent. Put your hands on your hips and tighten your gluts. As you bend your knees, lower your body in 2 counts. The second count brings your butt just above your knees. Now lift in 2 counts. The second count up brings you to your original

position. Each double-count up and double-count down is 1 rep. Do 8 reps to complete 1 set.

Plié with Pulses

Keeping your torso steady as you go down, pulse 3 times at the bottom of the move. After the third pulse, lift while squeezing your gluts.

Do 8 reps to complete 1 set.

Pliés

Do the regular plié: lower and lift your body, with your knees bending directly over your toes. On the lift, never lock your knees—keep them relaxed so that you keep the tension in your lower body muscles.

Do 8 reps to complete 1 set.

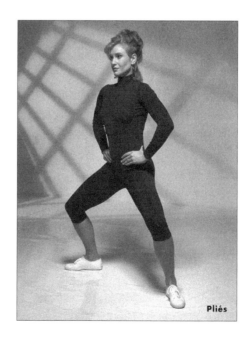

Pliés

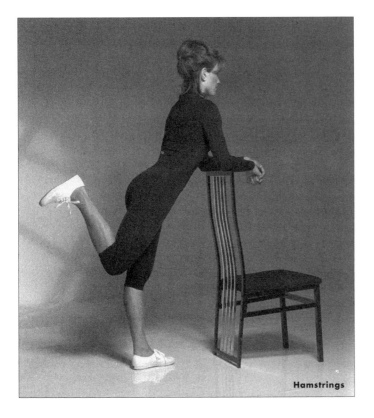

Hamstrings

Hamstrings

Go to your chair and stand a few feet behind the back of the chair. Rest your forearms on it for support. Stand with your weight on your left leg and your knee slightly bent. Extend your right leg behind you, keeping your knees together. Flex your foot and, in a continuous move, bend your knee and squeeze your hamstring as you lift your foot up toward your butt. Lower it to the original position.

Remember to contract your abs by exhaling on the lift and inhaling on the lowering of the leg.

Do 10 reps with your right leg to complete 1 set.

Hamstrings with Pulses

Now bring your right foot back up again, this time pulsing your foot 3 times at the top, getting your heel as close to your butt as you can. After 3 pulses at the top, lower your leg.

Do 10 reps with your right leg to complete 1 set.

Two-Count Hamstrings

Lift your right foot again—this time in a 2-count move. Lift halfway to the butt on the first count and then lift the rest of the way on count 2. Now lower halfway on 1 and lower back to the original position on the second count. This 2-count move is slower and more intense.

Do 10 reps with your right leg to complete 1 set.

Hamstrings/ Hamstrings with Pulses/Two-Count Hamstrings

Now switch legs and repeat the 3 hamstring sets with your left leg. Start by doing 1 set of 10 reps of the regular Hamstrings lift. Then do 1 set of 10 reps of the Hamstrings with Pulses lift. Finally, do 1 set of 10 reps of the Two-Count Hamstrings.

Four-Count Lunges

We're going to do the same Four-Count Lunges we introduced last week, but this week we're going to do more of them. Let's start with the right leg. Hold on to your chair with your left hand if you need help balancing, but if you can balance on your own, try it without your chair.

The counts are: (1) step, (2) press down, (3) push up, and (4) step back. Take a big step with your right leg and lower so that your butt is almost parallel to your knee. Your left leg, which is now extended behind you, also lowers. Be careful not to touch the floor with your left knee. Now, with your weight on your front (right) heel, push up and step back to your original position. Remember to keep your torso upright and neutral—your legs are doing all the work. Exhale when you lower down and push up.

Do 8 reps to complete 1 set on your right leg.

Let's switch working legs. Stand in the same place; keep your left hand on the chair and step forward with your left leg. Your right leg stays extended behind as you lower down, push up, and step back with your left leg.

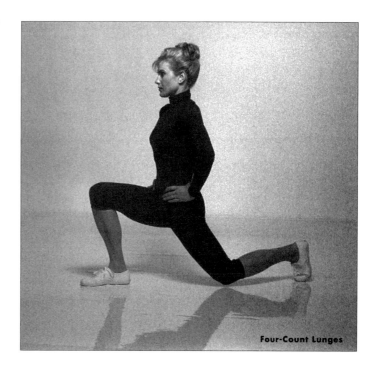

Four-Count Lunges

Do 1 set of 8 reps on your left leg.

For the last part of this exercise, do the Four-Count Lunge alternating right and left legs. It's right lunge, left lunge, and so on, for a total of 8 reps to complete 1 set.

Toe Taps

Back on both your feet, put your weight on your right leg and start tapping with your left foot.

Do 15 taps up and down, lifting your toes as high as you can.

Left-to-Right Taps

Now tap with your toes arcing to the left and then to the right.

Each right-to-left move counts as 1 rep. Do 15 reps with your left foot to complete 1 set.

Toe Taps/Left-to-Right Taps

Switch feet so that your weight is on your left leg and you tap with your right foot.

Do 15 regular Toe Taps to complete 1 set.

Do 15 Right-to-Left Taps to complete 1 set.

Repeat the sets with your left foot (15 Toe Taps and 15 Left-to-Right Taps) and then with your right foot (15 Toe Taps and 15 Right-to-Left Taps).

Now we're going to do a new form of calf raises.

Wrap-Leg Calf Raises

Standing on both legs and holding on to the back of the chair if you need help balancing, wrap the front of your left foot around your right calf, just above the ankle. Now work your calf muscle by raising and lowering your right heel 15 times.

Switch standing legs. This time wrap the front of your right foot around the left lower calf and raise and lower your left heel a total of 15 times.

Ready for the Calf Stretch?

Calf Stretch

Bring your right leg forward and bend it slightly at the knee. Your left leg will be behind you with your toes on the floor and your heel raised. Now press your left heel down against the floor. Bend your back knee, holding your heel down for 8 counts, stretching your left calf and soleus.

Let's switch working legs. Bring your left leg forward, bent slightly at the knee. Your right leg should be far enough behind you so that your right heel is lifted. Press your heel down onto the floor, bending your knee and stretching your right calf and soleus. Hold for 8 counts.

Time for the floor work, which is also different this week.

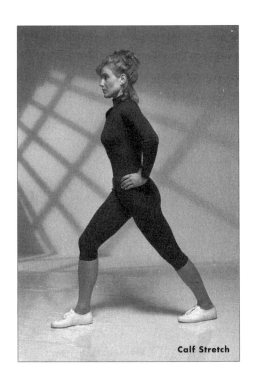

Calf Stretch

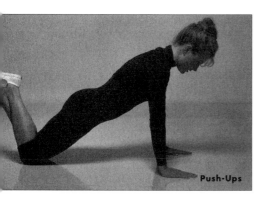
Push-Ups

Push-Ups

Get down on your hands and knees, with your arms straight, knees bent, and feet up, with the soles of your feet facing the ceiling. Cross your feet at the ankles. Place your hands on the floor, lined up with your shoulders.

Exhale as you push up with your arms. Tighten your abs and your butt as you lift. Make sure you don't arch your back—it should remain straight. Your head is forward, extended from your spine—not lifted or dropped.

Inhale as you lower your upper body back down but do not rest on the floor.

Do 3 sets of 8 reps.

Remember, if at any time you feel overburdened or if you feel you're getting out of good form—stop, rest, and start again.

Toe-to-Side Back Stretch

Lie down flat on the floor, on your stomach. Extend your arms and legs so your body is in a straight line. Inhale as you bring your right arm and left leg off the floor. Now turn your left foot out so your toes are pointing left. Exhale at the top and hold for a count of 8. Return to the original position.

Now switch so that your left arm and right leg are lifted off the floor. Point your foot out to the right side, working the side of your gluts along with your gluteus maximus. Hold the lift for a count of 8. Lower.

Get your chair close by. You're about to start supersetting.

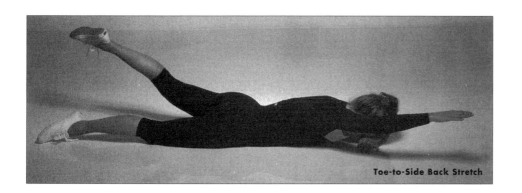
Toe-to-Side Back Stretch

SUPERSET:
Leg Extensions and Vertical Leg Raise

Leg Extension— Flexed

Sit on the floor, with your knees bent in front of you and your upper body resting on your elbows behind you. Place your hands under your lower back for support.

Start by straightening your left leg, lifting your foot from the floor but keeping your thighs together. Flex your foot. Remember to exhale on the lift so your abs pull in. Then lower your leg but don't touch the floor. Get ready to lift it again.

Do 5 reps with your left leg to complete 1 set.

Leg Extension— Toes Out

Now turn your foot so your toes are pointing out and do Leg Extensions on your left foot with your toes pointed to the left side. You're working the inner thigh.

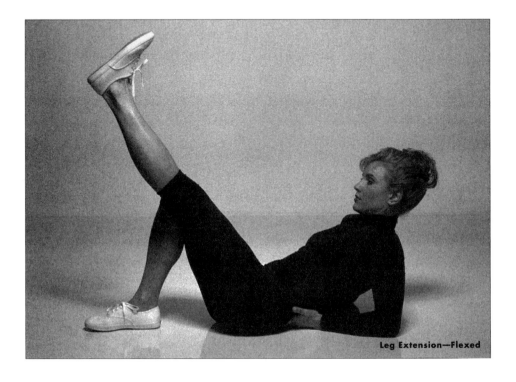

Leg Extension—Flexed

Do 5 reps with your left leg to complete 1 set.

Leg Extension—Toes In

Turn your toes in so they're pointed right. Lift and lower to work more of your outer thigh.

Do 5 reps with your left leg to complete 1 set.

Leg Extension—Flexed

Switch legs. Place your left leg back on the floor with a bent knee. Extend your right leg in front of you with your foot flexed and your toes pointed up.

Do 1 set of 5 reps with your right leg.

Leg Extension—Toes Out

Turn your right foot so your toes are pointing out to the right. Do 1 set of 5 reps with your toes pointed to the right.

Leg Extension—Toes In

Now turn your right foot in so it's pointed to your left.

Do 1 set of 5 reps with your foot pointed in.

Move over to your chair and get ready for leg raises.

Vertical Leg Raise

Still on the floor on your back, position yourself so your butt is in front of the chair seat. Your arms are at your sides and your hands are flat. Now place your feet and lower calves up on the chair seat. Your knees are bent.

Extend your left leg straight up. Now, digging your right heel into the chair, push up and squeeze your butt as you raise your (left) extended

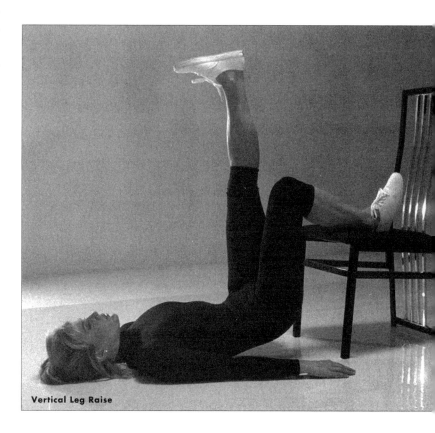

Vertical Leg Raise

leg higher and your butt comes up slightly off the floor. Keep your back flat on the floor. Lower your butt to the floor and get ready to push up again.

Do 2 sets of 8 reps with your left leg.

Immediately switch legs so that your left foot and calf are resting on the chair seat. Straighten your right leg. Push up with your left heel and raise your leg so your butt comes up off the floor. Squeeze your gluts as you raise up.

Do 2 sets of 8 reps with your right leg.

Now let's move on to your next superset.

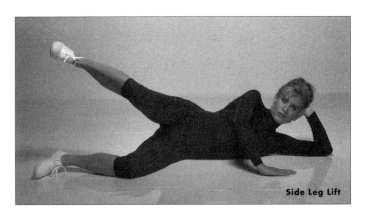

Side Leg Lift

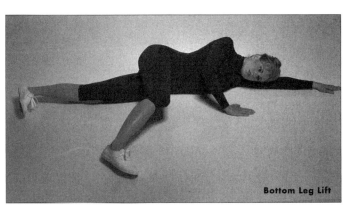

Bottom Leg Lift

SUPERSET:
Side Leg Lift and Bottom Leg Lift

Side Leg Lift with Pulses

Lie on your left side, with your hips stacked (not leaning forward or backward), knees bent slightly, and your legs together. Your left arm is bent at the elbow and your head is resting on your hand. Your right arm is in front of you, anchoring you in place.

Flex your right foot and raise your right leg without moving your upper body. When you get your leg up to the top, pulse 3 times by pushing up and lowering slightly before you lower your leg to the starting position. Do not rest your leg before you lift it again.

Do 2 sets of 20 reps with the right leg.

Bottom Leg Lift with Pulses

Stay in the same position as for Side Leg Lifts, but put your head down so it's resting on your extended left arm. Now flex your left foot and lift your (left) bottom leg, pulsing 3 times at the top by lifting and lowering slightly. Then lower your leg but do not rest it before you lift again.

Do 2 sets of 20 reps with the left leg.

Side Leg Lift with Pulses

Now switch sides so you're lying on your right side, hips stacked and knees bent slightly. Rest your head on your right hand.

Flex your left foot. Pulse it 3 times at the top before you lower it. Do not rest your leg before you lift it again.

Do 2 sets of 20 reps with the left leg.

Bottom Leg Lift with Pulses

Now put your right arm down and rest your head on your extended arm.

This time raise your right leg, with a flexed foot, and pulse it 3 times before you lower it.

Do 2 sets of 20 reps with your right leg.

Abdominals

Crunches with Pelvic Tilt

Lie on your back with your knees bent, and your hands behind your head. Keep your feet on the floor and tilt your pelvis as you lift your upper body toward your bent knees. Imagine your bottom rib and your hip bones coming closer together as you move. Lower your shoulders but don't rest at the bottom.

Do 1 set of 20 reps with the pelvic tilt.

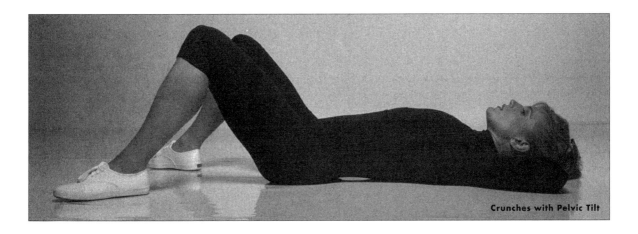

Crunches with Pelvic Tilt

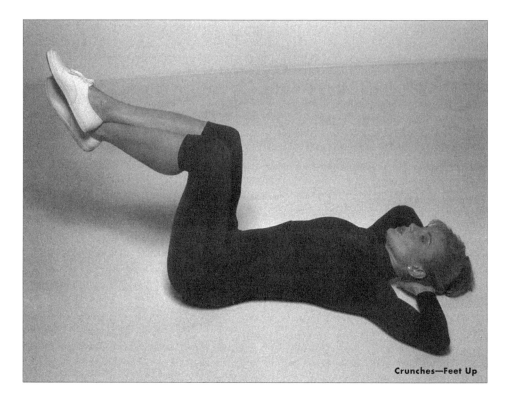

Crunches—Feet Up

Crunches—Feet Up

Now lift your knees so your legs form a right angle to your hips. Cross your feet at the ankles. Keep your hands behind your head and lift your torso up toward your bent knees. Exhale as you lift. Inhale as you lower but do not touch the floor with your shoulders.

Do 1 set of 10 reps with your feet and knees up in the air.

Crunches— Legs Straight Up

This time continue lifting your upper body but change your lower body movement. Beginning with your feet and knees still up in the air, straighten your legs. Now, lift your hips as you also lift your legs straight up. At the same time, raise your shoulders. As you lower your upper body, bring your legs back into the bent knee position with your knees at a right angle to your hips. Exhale as you lift and inhale as you lower.

Do 1 set of 20 reps of this move.

Crunches—Feet Up

Keep your feet and knees in the up and bent position.

Do 1 set of 10 reps of lifting your upper body to your raised knees.

Crunches—Hip Lift

Beginning with your feet and knees in the air, first straighten your legs. Place your hands under your hips. Lift your butt and legs straight up off the floor. Exhale on this exertion. Keep your legs in an imaginary tube so that you can't swing your legs forward as you work your lower abs with the lift. Your upper body stays flat on the floor. Bring your butt back down to the floor, keeping your legs vertical, and lift again.

Do 1 set of 10 reps and rest.

Do a second set of 10 reps and rest.

Do a third set of 10 reps and rest.

If you are strong enough, do 20 reps before you rest. If you're really advanced, do all 30 reps before you go on to the next set.

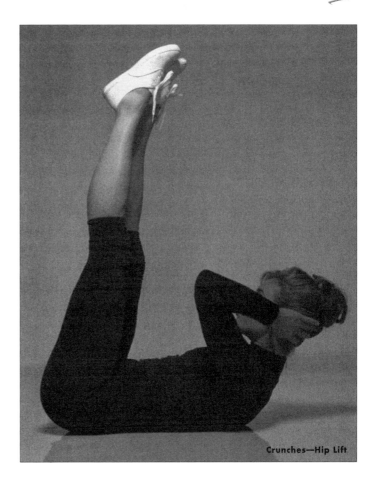

Crunches—Hip Lift

Crunches with Pelvic Tilt

Finish this abs segment with your feet on the floor, knees bent. Do a pelvic tilt as you bring your upper body up toward your knees.

Do 1 set of 10 reps.

Cool-Down

Now move on to the cool-down stretches, which begin on page 51.

Good work! Do this week's workout at least 4 times. You're going to feel very accomplished when you get through it. It's just a couple of weeks until you earn your star billing as a primetime body!

WEEK 4 SUMMARY

Exercise	Reps	Sets
Superset:		
Overhead Press	10	2
Biceps Curls—Angled	10	2
Superset:		
Triceps Extension—Palm Up	10 right/10 left	2
Rear Deltoids	10	2
Superset:		
Front Raise	10	2
Triceps Dips	10	2
Two-Count Pliés	8	1
Plié with Pulses	8	1
Pliés	8	1
Hamstrings	10 right/10 left	1
Hamstrings with Pulses	10 right/10 left	1
Two-Count Hamstrings	10 right/10 left	1
Four-Count Lunges	8 right/8 left/8 alternate	1
Toe Taps	15 right/15 left	2
Left-to-Right (and Right-to-Left) Taps	15 left/15 right	2
Wrap-Leg Calf Raises	15 right/15 left	1
Calf Stretch	hold 8 counts each side	1
Push-Ups	8	3
Toe-to-Side Back Stretch	hold 8 counts each side	1

WEEK 4 SUMMARY, CONTINUED

Exercise	Reps	Sets
Superset:		
Leg Extension—Flexed	5 right/5 left	1
Leg Extension—Toes Out	5 right/5 left	1
Leg Extension—Toes In	5 right/5 left	1
Vertical Leg Raise	8 right/8 left	2
Superset:		
Side Leg Lift with Pulses	20 right/20 left	2
Bottom Leg Lift with Pulses	20 right/20 left	2
Crunches with Pelvic Tilt	20	1
Crunches—Feet Up	10	1
Crunches—Legs Straight Up	20	1
Crunches—Feet Up	10	1
Crunches—Hip Lift	10 (rest after each set optional)	3
Crunches with Pelvic Tilt	10	1

8

Playing the Part

Week 5: Hitting Your Stride and Keeping It Fresh

Every time you push something, whether it's against the floor when you do push-ups, or against a door that you want to open, your muscles are actually pulling to do their work. We're pulling that you can push your way through these last two weeks of our program.

If you want to be successful at working out, you need to be able to do work in more ways than one. You need to find ways to keep your workout fresh.

It's easy to burn out on anything you do repeatedly, but it's important to repeat what you do if your success depends on repetition. Getting your body in shape and keeping it looking good depends entirely on your commitment to repeated performance.

Actors use imagination to help them act. Good actors look for some "flash" to connect them with their roles. Sometimes it comes in the form of a picture or from music. They find something that triggers their ability to connect with their role and construct it so their character comes alive, and stays alive for as long as they're performing.

That's what you have to do, too. The role you want to play is that of a woman whose body and whose attitude show she is in control of herself. Julianne Phillips, who has long been recognized as one of Hollywood's

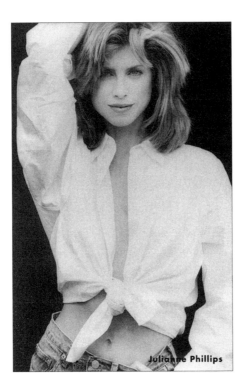

Julianne Phillips

fittest celebrities, says that working out improves your mental and physical self.

Another client, actress Elizabeth Berkley, got her first starring role in a major motion picture (*Showgirls*) in large part because she's a terrific dancer. But the fact that her great shape shows her character is in control of her life was just as important to the powers who chose her for this leading role. Working out gave Elizabeth the stamina to work 18-hour days, six days a week during filming. It also gave her the mental preparedness to meet the challenges of a difficult role.

Despite all their dedication to exercise and being in great shape, even Julianne and Elizabeth have to look for those sparks to keep them-

selves motivated. For Elizabeth, it's something as simple as reversing the way we count reps in the program. So instead of calling out 1-2-3-4-5, we count 5-4-3-2-1. For Julianne, it's the additional challenge from adding weights and mixing different exercise—so we mix in step-and-slide with upper and lower body moves.

Candice Bergen needs constant stimulation when she exercises. She's a perfect case-in-point when it comes to repetitious exercise. She doesn't like it. So we're always mixing up the program. We don't allow time for boredom to creep in. We do lots of supersets so we stay moving until the end of our workout. We always finish with stretching. Candice says the stretching increases her flexibility and it just plain makes her feel good.

Well, that's what we want you to feel, too. This week we're giving you what we give all our primetime bodies: change, challenge, and the chance to hit your stride. . . . Ready? 3-2-1-Go for it!

This Week's Plan

We have supersets again for you this week. Pay close attention because they are somewhat different from the moves we did last week. And watch for the number of reps. Many of them have changed again this week.

We hope that if you haven't used hand weights yet, you will start this week. If it's the cost of weights that is keeping you from using them, please consider using something you might already have around the house. You might want to try a full liter-size bottle of water in each hand or a large (about a pound and one-half) cylindrical container of kitchen cleanser in each hand. Just make sure the items you use can be easily grasped and balanced and that they are not slippery. They should be tightly closed to prevent leakage and they should be unbreakable.

Our directions this week do call for weights, but if you do not use weights, follow the same directions anyway because the moves will be the same.

Week 5

Warm-Up

Start your workout with a warm-up. By this week, you've gotten more accustomed to working out and you should be feeling a new and higher level of energy. If you haven't been doing a vigorous aerobic workout

before you start our program, try doing one this week: a brisk walk, a hike, a bike ride, or even dancing. The more calories you burn with aerobic activity, the faster you're going to see your primetime muscles!

Remember, the warm-up is going to help you burn calories, too. Add our warm-up to any other aerobic activity you do—or do ours alone. The key to a good performance is good preparation. So turn to page 17 for our warm-up and prepare to perform.

Now let's get right into our first superset.

SUPERSET:
Overhead Press and Hammerhead Curls

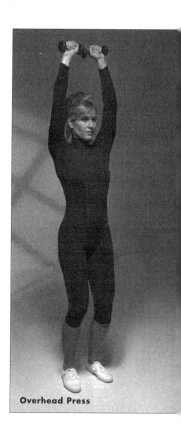

Overhead Press

Overhead Press

Stand in the basic position with your legs shoulder-width apart and your knees slightly bent. Let your arms hang down at your sides, with weights in your hands.

Moving only your arms, bend them up at the elbows with your palms facing forward. This is your starting position. Exhale as you lift your arms, straightening them completely as you lift overhead. Hold for a beat and inhale as you lower your arms to their starting position.

Do 12 reps to complete 1 set.

Hammerhead Curls

Start with your hands down at your sides. Still holding your weights, turn the palms of your hands to face each other. Now curl up your arms, aiming your thumbs toward your shoulders. Exhale and squeeze on

the lift and slowly lower your hands back down to starting position.

Do 12 reps to complete 1 set.

Overhead Press

Now go back to the Overhead Press. Start with your elbows bent and your hands at shoulder level—your palms facing forward. Lift your arms until they're fully extended; hold and lower.

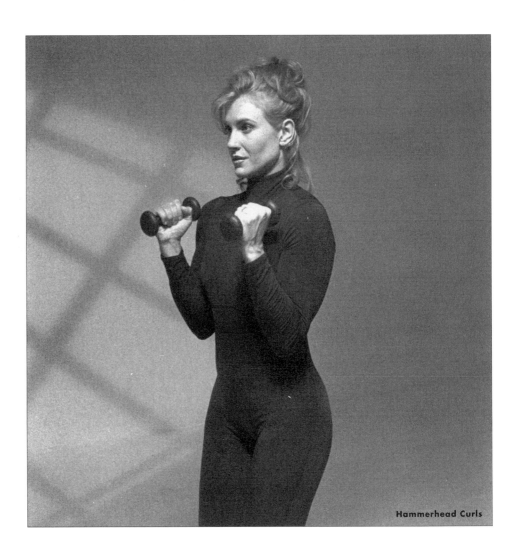

Hammerhead Curls

Do 12 reps to complete 1 set and then repeat the Hammerhead Curls.

Hammerhead Curls

Start with your hands down at your sides, palms facing in toward each other. Squeeze your biceps as you lift so your thumbs come up toward your shoulders. Lower.

Do 12 reps to complete 1 set.

SUPERSET:
Rear Deltoids and Triceps Extension

Rear Deltoids

Sit on the edge of your chair. Bend forward at the waist and, with a weight in each hand, lift your arms out to the sides. Bring them up to shoulder level and squeeze your shoulder blades together. Remember to keep your wrists steady and do not let your head drop. Bring your arms back down so your knuckles are once again facing the floor. Exhale on the lift.

Do 12 reps to complete 1 set. Immediately start the next exercise.

Triceps Extension— Palm Up

Stand by your chair and place your left knee on the seat. Your right leg is straight, with your knee slightly bent. Lean forward from the waist so that your upper body is parallel to the chair seat. Make sure your back is flat.

With a weight in your right hand, bring your right arm up so it is even with your back, and bend your elbow. This is your starting position. Extend your forearm, squeezing your triceps as you lift, and turn your palm up to the ceiling. Return to the starting position.

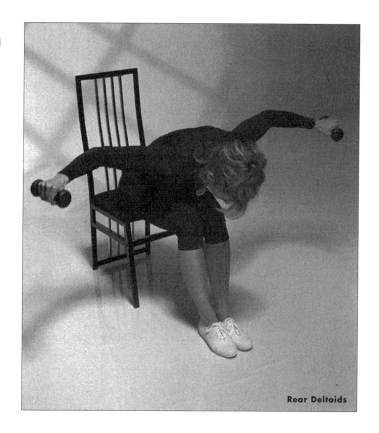

Rear Deltoids

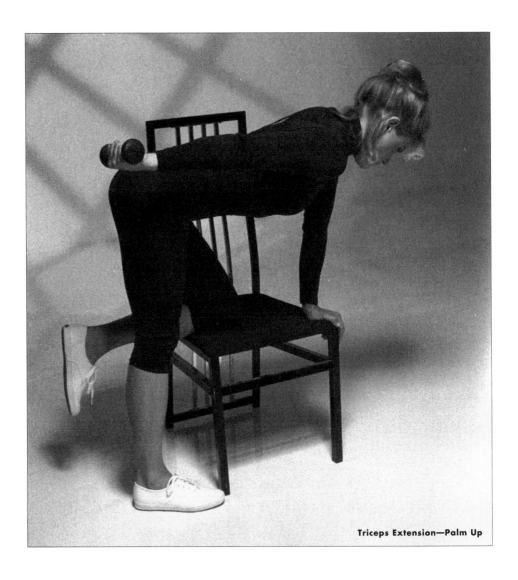

Triceps Extension—Palm Up

Do 12 reps with your right arm to complete 1 set and go right back to sitting on the edge of your chair.

Rear Deltoids

Do 12 reps to complete 1 set. Return to your standing position, ready to work your left triceps.

Triceps Extension— Palm Up

Place your right knee on the seat of the chair. Your left leg should be straight, with your knee slightly bent. Your weight is in your left hand. Bend your upper body over the chair seat, keeping a flat back.

Raise your left arm, elbow bent, so that your upper arm is even with your back. Now extend your forearm, squeezing your triceps as you lift and turning your palm up toward the ceiling. Return to the starting position.

Do 12 reps with your left arm to complete 1 set. Let's move on to the next superset.

SUPERSET:

Front Raise and Triceps Dips

Front Raise

Back to standing in your basic position with your knees slightly bent

and your weights in both hands, exhale as you lift your arms straight out in front of you. Bring them to shoulder height, palms facing down. Inhale, and slowly lower your arms, controlling their move against the weight of gravity.

Do 12 reps to complete 1 set. Go right to the chair.

Triceps Dips

Sit on the edge of the chair with your hands on the front edge of the seat and your legs out in front of you, knees bent. Start with your butt at chair-seat level and dip down so that your butt and your back skim the chair as you lower. Exhale as you lift back up.

Do 12 reps to complete 1 set.

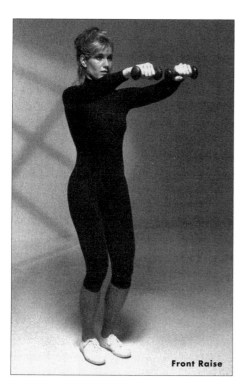

Front Raise

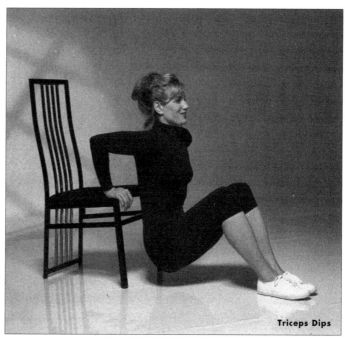

Triceps Dips

Front Raise/ Triceps Dips

In your standing position, do a second set of 12 Front Raises.

Return to the chair and do a second set of 12 Tricep Dips.

Let's move on to working your lower body.

Three-Count Pliés

This week we add a count to the downward motion, so get into position with your feet on the 10 and 2 spots of your imaginary clock. Bend your knees slightly and place your hands on your hips.

Tighten your gluts as you bend your knees, lowering your body in 3 counts. Each count moves you a little lower, with the third count bringing your butt almost even with your knees. Now lift in 1 count to the original position.

Do 8 reps to complete 1 set. Then lower your body for Plié with Pulses.

Plié with Pulses

Keeping your torso steady as you go down, pulse 3 times at the bottom of the move. After the third pulse, lift up to the original position by squeezing your gluts.

Do 8 reps to complete 1 set.

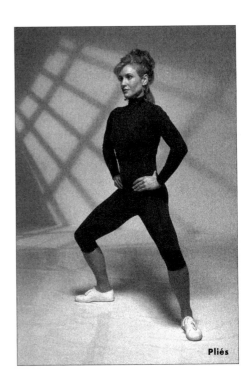

Pliés

Pliés

Now do single pliés. Remember, do not come all the way up and straighten your knees completely. Keep them relaxed so you can keep the tension in your lower body muscles.

Do 8 reps to complete 1 set.

Four-Count Lunges

We're adding more reps to the Four-Count Lunges. Let's start with your right leg.

Hold on to your chair with your left hand if you need balancing. If you don't need the chair, do the lunges with your arms out to the side to help you balance.

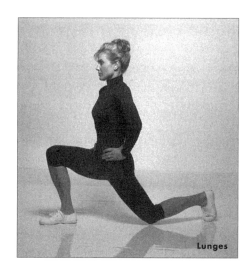
Lunges

and lift your right leg, with foot flexed. Extend it behind you and, in the same motion, bend it at the knee and squeeze your hamstrings as you lift your heel up toward your butt. Lower it to your original position.

Do 10 reps with your right leg.

Hamstrings with Pulses

Now repeat the same move, but at the top, pulse your leg 3 times and then lower it.

Do 10 reps with your right leg.

The counts are: (1) step, (2) press down, (3) push up, and (4) step back.

Take a big step out in front of you with your right leg and leave your left leg back. Now bend your knees as you lower, bringing your butt down to knee level. Putting your weight on your right heel, push up and step back with your right leg to the original position.

Do 10 reps on your right leg.

Switch legs by stepping forward with your left leg, leaving your right leg behind you, bending both knees as you lower your butt down to knee level.

Do 10 reps with the left leg to complete 1 set.

Hamstrings

Stand behind the back of your chair, holding on to it for support. Stand with your weight on your left leg

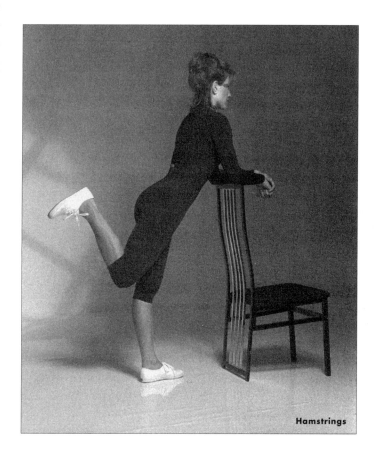
Hamstrings

Two-Count Hamstrings

Lift your right foot again—this time in a 2-count move. Lift your foot toward your butt in 2 counts. Then lower in 2 counts.

Do 10 reps with your right leg to complete 1 set.

Hamstrings/ Hamstrings with Pulses/Two-Count Hamstrings

Now switch legs and repeat the hamstring group with your left leg.

Do 10 reps of the regular Hamstrings lift. Do 10 reps of the Hamstrings with Pulses.

Finish with 10 reps of the Two-Count Hamstrings.

Stand in the basic position and get ready for Toe Taps.

Toe Taps

With your weight on your right leg, start tapping with your left foot. Flex your foot as high as you can and tap down.

Do 15 reps with your left foot.

Left-to-Right Taps

Follow with taps out to the left and right. Count each left-to-right arc as 1 rep.

Do 15 reps with your left foot to complete 1 set.

Toe Taps/ Left-to-Right Taps

Switch feet. Put your weight on your left leg and tap with your right foot.

Do 15 regular taps with your right foot.

Follow with 15 taps from right to left with your right foot.

Repeat the set with your left foot (15 Toe Taps and 15 Left-to-Right Taps) and then again with your right foot (15 Toe Taps and 15 Right-to-Left Taps).

Wrap-Leg Calf Raise

You may need to hold on to the back of your chair for balance on this exercise. Standing straight on both legs to begin, wrap the front of your left foot around your right calf, just above the ankle. Now raise and lower your right heel 15 times.

Switch legs. Wrap your right foot around your left calf. Raise and lower your left heel 15 times.

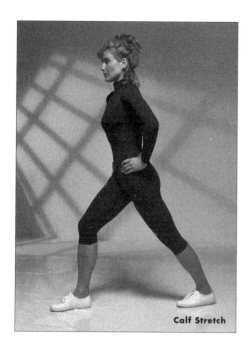

Calf Stretch

the floor, stretching your left calf. Hold for 8 counts.

Switch legs. Bring your left leg forward and keep your right leg back, with your toes on the floor and your heel raised. Press your right heel down into the floor and stretch your right calf for a count of 8.

Push-Ups—Elbows In

We're changing the form a little this week to work more of your triceps—and we're adding reps.

Get down on your hands and knees, extend your arms, and bend your knees so that the soles of your feet are facing the ceiling. Cross your feet at the ankles.

Lower your body so your hands are right next to your chest (rather than near your shoulders, as before)

Calf Stretch

Bring your right leg forward and bend it slightly at the knee. Keep your left leg back, with your toes on the floor and your heel raised. Now press your left heel down on

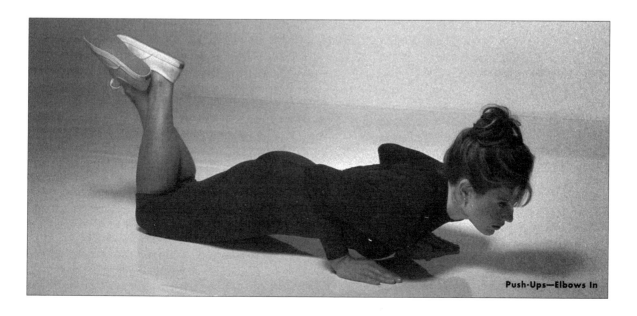

Push-Ups—Elbows In

and your elbows are right in to your sides. Now push up with your arms, tightening your butt and your abs as you lift. Make sure your back stays flat, your head is extended straight out from the top of your spine (not lifted or dropped), and your fingers are facing forward. Do not rest on the floor between push-ups. Remember, if at any time you feel yourself getting out of good form or too weak to continue, stop, rest, and start again.

Do 3 sets of 10 reps.

Toe-to-Side Back Stretch

Lying on your stomach, extend your arms and legs so your body is in a straight line. Raise your right arm and left leg off the floor, stretching outward as far as you can. Turn your left foot out so your toes point to the left. Hold for a count of 8. Return your arm and leg to the floor.

Now lift your left arm and right leg off the floor, stretching as far as you can. Turn your right foot out so your toes point to the right. Hold for a count of 8. Return your arm and leg to the floor.

SUPERSET:
Side Leg Lift with Pulses, Vertical Leg Raise, and Bottom Leg Lift

This set is a super challenge. We start with the abduction, for the outer thighs.

Side Leg Lift with Pulses

Lie on your left side, with hips stacked straight, knees bent slightly, and your legs together. Bend your left arm at the elbow and rest your head on your left hand. Place your

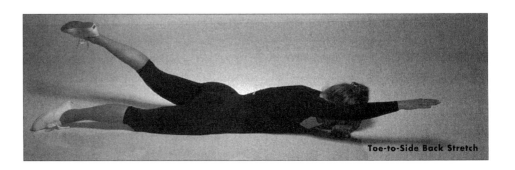

Toe-to-Side Back Stretch

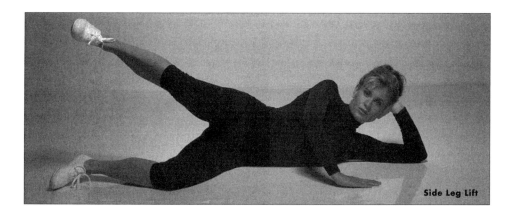

Side Leg Lift

right arm in front of you, anchoring you so you don't tilt back.

Now flex your right foot and lift your leg up without tilting backward. At the top, pulse your leg 3 times. Lower your leg in 1 count.

Do 15 reps with your right leg to complete 1 set. Immediately get into position for Vertical Leg Raises.

Vertical Leg Raise

Lie on your back and place your right leg up on your chair so that your foot and your calf are resting on the chair. Extend your left leg straight up and place your hands on the floor at your sides. Now, digging into the chair with your right heel and keeping your left leg vertical, lift your butt off the floor, squeezing your gluts as you raise up. Do not lift your back off the floor. Bring your butt down but do not rest it before you raise it up again.

Do 10 reps with your left leg to complete 1 set.

Bottom Leg Lift

Roll over onto your right side and bring your left leg over in front of your body. Rest your head on your extended arm. Flex your bottom (right) foot and lift your leg to work the adductor, or inner thigh.

Do 15 reps with your right leg to complete 1 set.

Now let's do the whole superset again on the other side.

Side Leg Lift with Pulses

Lie on your right side with your hips stacked straight, your knees bent slightly, and legs together. Your head is supported with your right hand and your left arm is in front of you, anchoring your body.

Now lift your left leg up and pulse it 3 times. Lower it in 1 count.

Do 15 reps with your left leg to complete 1 set.

Vertical Leg Raise

Still on the floor, place your left calf on the chair seat and raise your right leg straight in the air. Press into the chair with your left heel, squeeze your gluts, and lift your butt off the floor, keeping your back flat on the floor. Lower, but do not rest on the floor between lifts.

Do 10 reps with your right leg to complete 1 set.

Bottom Leg Lift

Now roll over onto your left side and extend your arm flat, resting your head on your arm. Place your right leg in front of your body. Lift up your bottom (left) leg with your foot flexed. Do 15 reps with your left leg and get ready to work on your:

Abdominals

Three-count pulses will be in all the abs exercises this week. If you can, we'd like you to do all the abs work without stopping. But if you don't feel strong enough or if you feel you're getting out of good form—stop, rest, and start again.

Start on your back, hands behind your head, knees bent, and feet flat on the floor. Remember to exhale at the top of each lift so that your abs are pulling in when you lift to your highest point and when you are pulsing.

Three-Count Crunches with Pulses

Now lift up your upper body in 3 counts, pulling in on your abs as you lift. Lower in 1 count.

Do 10 reps to complete 1 set.

Pulses

Lower to your original position. Lift your upper body off the floor and pulse 10 times at the top of the lift. Lower.

Three-Count Crunches—Feet Up—with Pulses

Bring your knees and your feet up in the air and cross your feet at the ankles. Do a 3-count lift to your knees and lower your upper body.

Do 10 reps to complete 1 set.

Pulses

Now lift and pulse 10 times at the top. Lower.

Three-Count Crunches—Feet Up—Elbow to Knee

Your knees and feet are still up in the air and your feet are crossed at the ankles. Now as you lift in 3 counts, bring your right elbow toward your left knee. Come back down, with your upper body centered, in 1 count.

Do 10 reps with your right elbow to complete 1 set.

Now switch so that your left elbow comes up toward your right knee. Lift in 3 counts and return your upper body centered, so your chin is pointing between your knees. Lower in 1 count.

Do 10 reps with your left elbow to complete 1 set.

Three-Count Crunches—Legs Straight Up

Place your hands under your hips and bring your legs straight up. Raise your butt and legs in 3 counts, while your lower body stays flat on the floor.

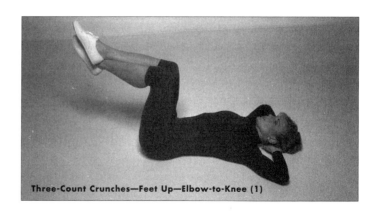

Three-Count Crunches—Feet Up—Elbow-to-Knee (1)

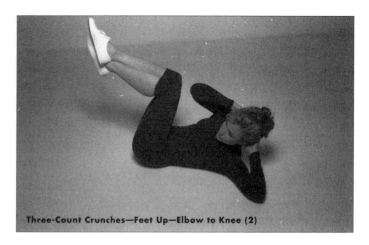

Three-Count Crunches—Feet Up—Elbow to Knee (2)

Do 10 reps to complete 1 set.

Cool-Down

Now move on to the cool-down stretches, which begin on page 51.

You're doing great. There's only one more week in our primetime bodies program and we suggest you sit down right now with your date book and schedule your four appointments with us next week.

We know from experience that if you've made it this far, getting to next week should be a piece of cake—non-fat, of course!

WEEK 5 SUMMARY

Exercise	Reps	Sets
Superset:		
Overhead Press	12	2
Hammerhead Curls	12	2
Superset:		
Rear Deltoids	12	2
Triceps Extension—Palm Up	12	2
Superset:		
Front Raise	12	2
Triceps Dips	12	2
Three-Count Pliés	8	1
Plié with Pulses	8	1
Pliés	8	1
Four-Count Lunges	10 right/10 left	1
Hamstrings	10 right/10 left	1
Hamstrings with Pulses	10 right/10 left	1
Two-Count Hamstrings	10 right/10 left	1
Toe Taps	15 right/15 left	2
Left-to-Right (and Right-to-Left) Taps	15 left/15 right	2
Wrap-Leg Calf Raise	15 right/15 left	1
Calf Stretch	hold 8 counts each side	
Push-Ups—Elbows In	10	3
Toe-to-Side Back Stretch	hold 8 counts each side	
Superset:		
Side Leg Lift with Pulses	15 right/15 left	1
Vertical Leg Raise	10 right/10 left	1
Bottom Leg Lift	15 right/15 left	1
Three-Count Crunches with Pulses	10	1
Pulses	10	1
Three-Count Crunches— Feet Up—with Pulses	10	1
Pulses	10	1
Three-Count Crunches— Feet Up—Elbow to Knee	10 right/10 left	1
Three-Count Crunches— Legs Straight Up	10	1

9

Producing Results

Week Six: The Pay-Off Is Big

It's the sixth and final week of our primetime bodies program. It's the week that's going to work you the hardest and make your muscles their sleekest yet, and it's the week that should swell your ego.

We know it's a challenge to do Push-Ups, Triceps Dips, Leg Raises, Lunges, and almost any move that makes your muscles stronger by overloading them. But very little that's worth achieving comes without hard work. And when you tackle it, it's worth shouting about—even if you shout while you're in the middle of it.

The leg work you're doing in our program is the same as we do with Ellen DeGeneres. Ellen hadn't been used to doing this kind of leg work when we started but she was supermotivated and consistently worked hard at building her endurance.

Though the road was rough and Ellen struggled at times, the closest to complaining we heard from her was a humorous crack about what she had gotten herself into. We began to wonder whether she was somehow different from everybody else when it comes to pain. After all, we've been working out for a while and we still shout and groan.

Finally, one day we asked her how she could remain so stoic. She admitted she hadn't wanted to let us think she couldn't do the work. But once she realized it was normal for everyone to experience some pain, she even screamed a couple of times. Of course, she never stops joking, but Ellen is serious about getting results.

Since you've made it this far, we think you're serious, too. So this week, we're giving you a workout that we believe will challenge you at the same time it keeps you interested. It's a workout we hope you will want to keep doing after this week as well. It's a workout that might make you scream but when it's all over it will definitely make you shout with pride.

The Action Returns

We have bigger supersets and more reps for you in the grand finale week. Our upper body exercises all call for hand weights and we hope you will be using them—whether they're the standard kind or your own version (see Chapter 8).

We hope you won't have much difficulty getting through our workout by now. But our standard rule still applies: if at any time you feel you're getting out of good form or that the work is too hard—stop, rest, and start again.

Week 6

Warm-Up

If you've been walking for your aerobic warm-up until now, why don't you try hiking this week? If you've been biking, how about adding some miles? If you've been doing our primetime warm-up, add some jumping jacks or do some extra sets of marching in place. When you try a little harder, you get a lot closer to achieving your goal of having a primetime body.

Our warm-up is on page 17.

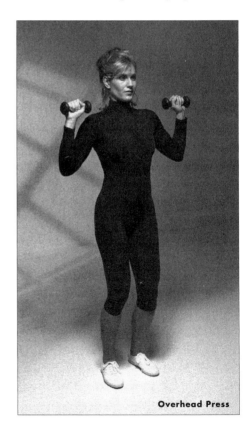

Overhead Press

SUPERSET:

Overhead Press, Triceps Dips, and Biceps Curls—Angled/Hammerhead Curls

Overhead Press

Start by standing in the basic position, legs shoulder-width apart and knees slightly bent. Bend your arms up at the elbows with your palms facing forward. Hold a weight in each hand.

Now lift your arms up overhead. Hold for a beat and lower your arms to the starting position.

Do 15 reps to complete 1 set. Move over to your chair and get ready for Triceps Dips.

Triceps Dips

Sit on the edge of your chair and place your hands on the front edge of the seat. Put your legs out in front of you, knees bent. Bend your elbows back slightly and keep your fingers forward.

Lift your butt out to chair-seat level, and dip down so your butt and back skim the chair as you lower. Exhale and lift back up. (Optimally, you'll lower far enough

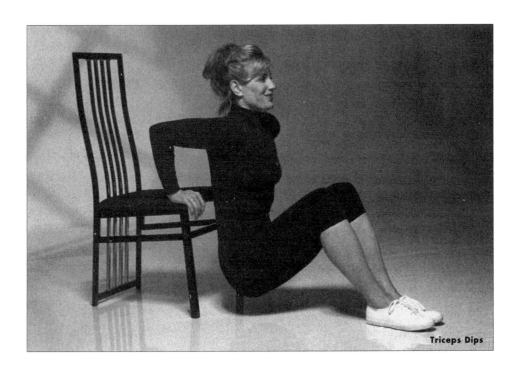

Triceps Dips

to get your elbows parallel with your shoulders.)

Do 15 reps to complete 1 set.

Biceps Curls— Angled

Stand in the basic position with your arms at your sides and hands holding weights, palms facing outward but angled slightly inward. Bend your arms at the elbow, squeezing your biceps as you curl up the weights at a 45-degree angle so that your palms and weights wind up facing each other on opposite sides of your chest.

Do 15 reps to complete 1 set.

Overhead Press

Do 15 reps of the Overhead Press and go back to the chair.

Triceps Dips

Do 15 reps of Triceps Dips and then stand with your weights.

Hammerhead Curls

Again in basic position, hold a weight in each hand with the palms of your hands facing in. Start with your hands down at your sides and curl up your arms, squeezing your biceps. Aim your thumbs toward

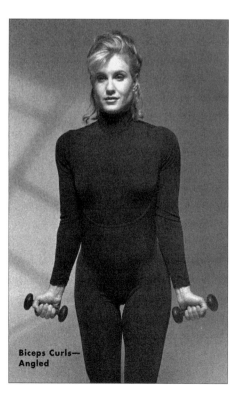

Biceps Curls—
Angled

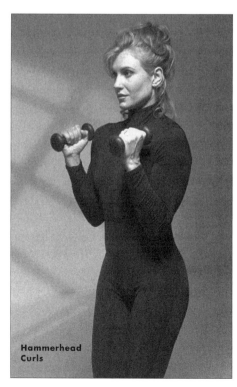

Hammerhead
Curls

your shoulders and lower your hands slowly, controlling the pull of the weights.

Do 15 reps to complete 1 set. Go back to the chair for your next superset.

SUPERSET:
Rear Deltoids and Front Raise

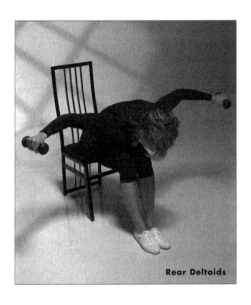

Rear Deltoids

Front Raise

Still holding a weight in each hand, exhale as you lift your straight arms up and out in front of you. Bring them to shoulder height, palms facing down. Inhale while you slowly lower your arms, controlling them against the pull of the weights.

Do 15 reps to complete 1 set. Go back to the chair.

Rear Deltoids

Sit on the edge of your chair and hold a weight in each hand. Bend forward at the waist and lift your arms out to your sides, bringing them up to shoulder level. Squeeze your shoulder blades together, keeping your wrists steady and bringing your arms back down so your knuckles are facing the floor.

Do 15 reps to complete 1 set.

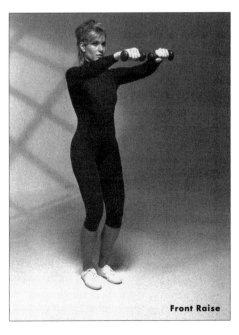

Front Raise

Rear Deltoids

Do 15 reps to complete this set and return to your standing position for your second set of the:

Front Raise

Do 15 reps to complete your second set and your second superset.

Triceps Extension— Palm Up

At the chair again, place your left knee on the seat. Your right leg is straight with a relaxed knee. Bend forward from the waist so that your upper body is over the chair seat. Make sure your back is flat.

With a weight in your right hand, bring your upper arm up so it is even with your back. Your elbow is bent so your hand is down, knuckles facing the floor.

Lift your forearm so that it is even with your back. Squeeze your triceps when you lift, and turn your palm up to the ceiling. Return your arm to the starting position.

Do 2 sets of 15 reps with your right arm. Then switch sides.

Place your right knee on the seat. Your left leg is straight with a relaxed knee. Bend forward from the waist. With a weight in your left hand, your upper arm even with your back, and your forearm hanging down at a right angle, lift your forearm. Squeeze your triceps as you lift, and turn your palm up toward the ceiling. Return to the starting position.

Do 2 sets of 15 reps with your left arm.

SUPERSET:
Pliés and Lunges

Stand with your feet on the 10 and 2 spots of an imaginary clock. Bend your knees slightly and put your hands on your hips.

Three-Count Pliés

Tighten your gluts and bend your knees. Lower in 3 counts. On the

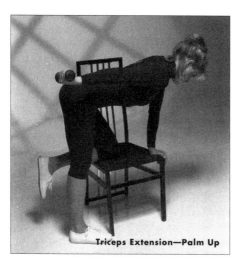

Triceps Extension—Palm Up

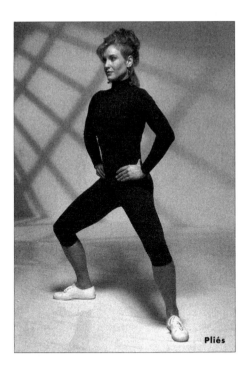

Pliés

Plié with Pulses

Now finish the plié with 8 reps of the Plié with Pulses.

Two-Count Lunges

Blend the moves from the Four-Count Lunge (see p. 114) into two counts. Step your right leg forward and bend at the knee for count 1; push back up and into the starting position with legs together for count 2.

Do 8 reps with your right leg.

Follow with your left leg. Step your left leg forward and bend at the knee for count 1; push back up into starting position for count 2.

Do 8 reps with your left leg.

Now alternate legs, starting with your right leg forward, then your left leg forward. Do 8 reps on alternating legs to complete the set and the superset.

third count, your butt should be almost even with your knees. Lift up in 1 count but do not straighten your knees completely—keep the tension on your inner thigh and glut muscles.

Do 8 reps of these Three-Count Pliés.

Plié with Pulses

Lower for the plié and when your butt is just above knee level, pulse 3 times. Lift.

Do 8 reps of the Plié with Pulses.

Pliés

Do 8 reps of the regular plié: lower in 1 move and lift in 1 move.

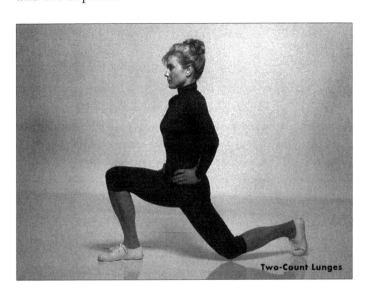

Two-Count Lunges

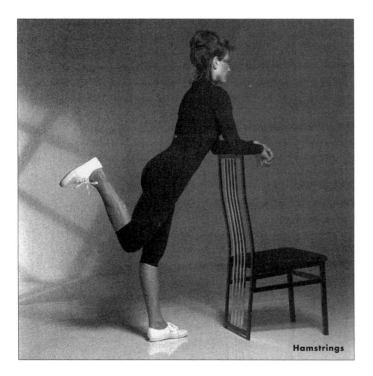

Hamstrings

Three-Count Hamstrings

Now do a 3-count lift. Lift your right heel toward your butt in 3 counts, moving it a little closer with each count. Then lower it in 1 count.

Do 10 reps with your right leg.

Hamstrings/ Hamstrings with Pulses/Three-Count Hamstrings

Now switch legs and repeat the same pattern with your left leg.

Do 10 reps of the regular Hamstrings.

Do 10 reps of the Hamstrings with Pulses.

Finish with 10 reps of the Three-Count Hamstrings.

Hamstrings

Stand behind the back of your chair, holding on for support. Stand with your weight on your left leg and lift your right leg. Flex your right foot. Extend your leg behind you and bend your knee. Squeeze your hamstrings as you lift your heel up toward your butt. Lower it to your original position.

Do 10 reps with your right leg.

Toe Taps

Rest your weight on your right leg and tap with your left foot.

Do 20 taps with your left foot.

Hamstrings with Pulses

Lift your right heel up again, but at the top, pulse your leg 3 times and then lower it.

Do 10 reps with your right leg.

Left-to-Right Taps

Follow with 15 taps with your left foot, arcing to the left and right. Each left-to-right move is 1 rep.

Toe Taps/Left-to-Right Taps

Switch feet. Lean your weight on your left leg and tap with your right foot.

Do 20 Toe Taps.

Follow with 15 Right-to-Left Taps.

Repeat the sets with your left foot.

Do 20 Toe Taps.

Do 15 Left-to-Right Taps.

Repeat the sets with your right foot.

Do 20 Toe Taps.

Do 15 Right-to-Left Taps.

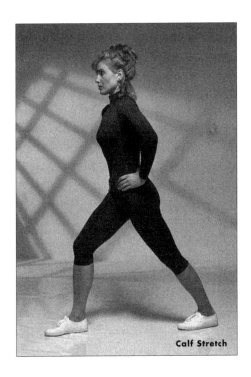

Calf Stretch

Wrap-Leg Calf Raise

Standing up straight on both legs, wrap the front of your left foot around your right calf, just above the ankle.

Raise and lower your right heel 15 times.

Switch standing legs. Wrap your right foot around your left lower calf.

Raise and lower your left heel 15 times.

Calf Stretch

Bring your right leg forward and bend it slightly at the knee. Leave your left leg back, keeping your toes on the floor and raising your heel. Now press your left heel down on the floor, stretching your left calf. Hold for 8 counts.

Switch legs. Bring your left leg forward and leave your right leg back, keeping your toes on the floor and raising your heel. Press the right heel down on the floor and stretch your right calf for a count of 8.

Push-Ups— Elbows In

Down on your hands and knees, extend your arms and bend your knees so that the soles of your feet are facing the ceiling. Cross your feet at the ankles.

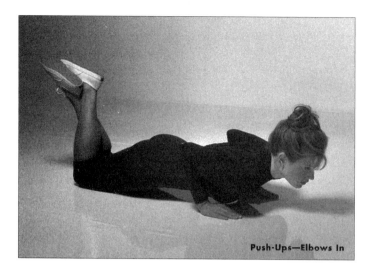

Push-Ups—Elbows In

Toe-to-Side Back Stretch

Lie flat on your stomach and extend your arms and legs so your body forms a straight line. Lift your right arm and left leg off the floor. Turn your left foot out so your toes are pointing out to the left. Now stretch that arm and leg and hold for a count of 8. Return your right arm and left leg to the floor.

Bring your left arm and right leg off the floor. Turn your right foot out to the side and stretch your arm and leg as far as you can. Hold for a count of 8. Return your left arm and right leg to the floor.

Place your hands right next to your chest so that when you are lowered your elbows are right next to your sides. Lower with your arms and do not rest on the floor. Tighten your butt and your abs as you lift. Make sure your back stays flat and your head is extended straight out from the top of your spine. Your fingers face forward.

Do 3 sets of 15 reps.

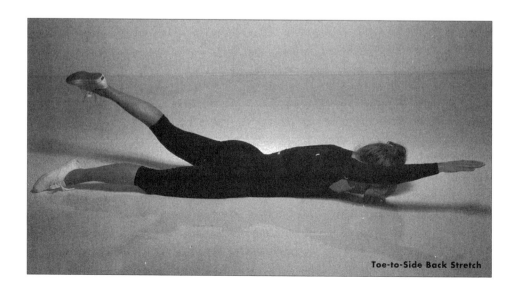

Toe-to-Side Back Stretch

SUPERSET:

Side Leg Lift—Knee to Chest/Vertical Leg Raises/Bottom Leg Lift with Pulses

Side Leg Lift— Knee to Chest

We have a different abduction move for you this week. Lie on your left side, with your hips stacked straight and your head supported with your left hand. Bend your knees, flex your foot, and support your upper body with your right arm in front of you.

Now raise your top leg a few inches; this is your starting position. Bring your knee in toward your chest, then extend your leg back out in a straight line with your upper body, all the while feeling the tension in your top outer thigh.

Do 15 reps with your right leg to complete 1 set. Now turn onto your back.

Vertical Leg Raise

Bend your right leg and place your foot and calf on your chair seat. Lift

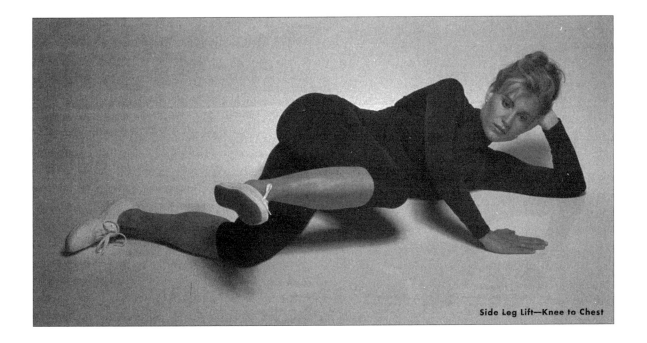

Side Leg Lift—Knee to Chest

your left leg straight up and place your hands at your sides.

Dig in to the chair with your right heel and lift your butt off the floor, squeezing your gluts as you lift. Do not lift your back. Bring your butt back down but do not rest it between raises.

Do 10 reps with your left leg.

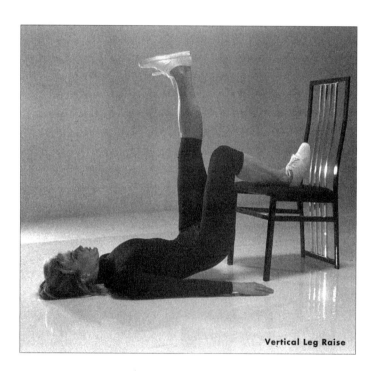

Vertical Leg Raise

Vertical Leg Raise with Pulses

Now we're adding another move, so stay where you are and squeeze your gluts while you lift your left leg again. This time pulse 3 times at the top.

Do 10 reps with your left leg and turn away from the chair to work your adductor.

Bottom Leg Lift with Pulses

Lie on your right side with your hips and legs stacked straight and your head resting on your right extended arm. Flex your right foot and bring your left arm and top leg in front of your body for support.

Lift your bottom leg and pulse it 3 times at the top. Lower in 1 count but do not rest it on the floor between lifts.

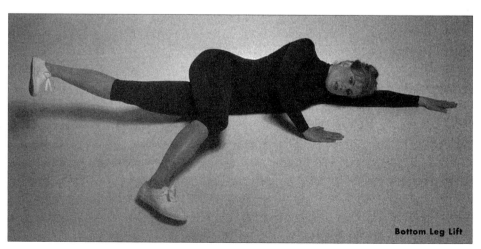

Bottom Leg Lift

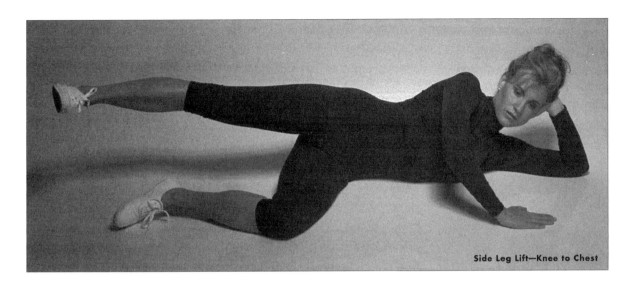

Side Leg Lift—Knee to Chest

Do 15 reps with the right leg.

Stay where you are. We're going to repeat this whole superset with the other legs this time.

Side Leg Lift— Knee to Chest

Bring your head back up and rest it on your right hand. Bend your knees, raise your top leg, and bring the knee in toward your chest. Extend it back out straight, in line with your upper body. Remember, keep it lifted but do not tilt your body back— you're working against gravity.

Do 15 reps with the left leg and go back to the chair.

Vertical Leg Raise

Place your left foot and calf on the chair and extend your right leg straight up. Rest your hands at your sides. Lift your butt off the floor by digging your left heel into the chair and squeezing your gluts. Lower but do not rest on the floor between lifts. Remember to keep your back flat on the floor.

Do 10 reps with the right leg and stay right where you are.

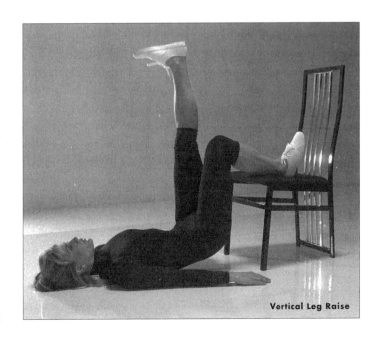

Vertical Leg Raise

Vertical Leg Raise with Pulses

Continue lifting and, at the top, pulse 3 times. Lower in 1 count.

Do 10 reps with the right leg.

Come off the chair and back onto your left side.

Bottom Leg Lift with Pulses

Lie on your left side, with your hips and legs stacked straight and your head resting on your extended arm. Flex your left foot and bring your left arm and your top leg forward. Lift your bottom leg and pulse it 3 times at the top. Then lower in 1 count but do not rest it on the floor between lifts. Remember, do not let your body tilt back.

Do 15 reps with the left leg and go back to your chair.

Abdominals

Crunches with Chair

Place both your feet and calves on the seat of the chair. Your upper body is flat on the floor, at a right angle to your quads. Place your hands behind your head.

Now lift your torso up toward your quads. It's very important to exhale and pull in your abs here. Do not rest your upper body on the floor between lifts.

Do 20 reps to complete 1 set.

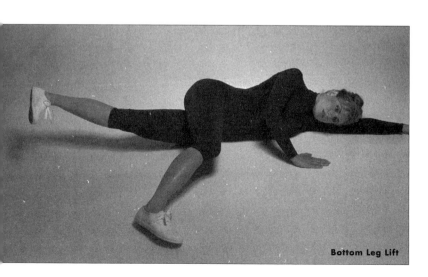

Bottom Leg Lift

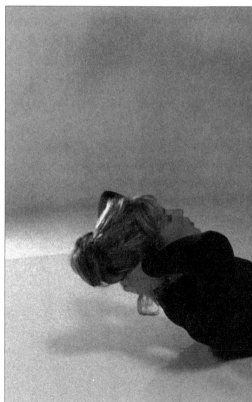

Crunches with Chair—Elbow to Knee

Now place your right hand on the back of your right thigh. Pull your right knee in slightly toward your chest. Lift with your left shoulder and elbow pointing up to your right knee. Remember, do not twist your spine and do not pull on your head or neck—use your abs to pull you up. Exhale on the lift.

Do 20 reps with your left elbow to complete 1 set.

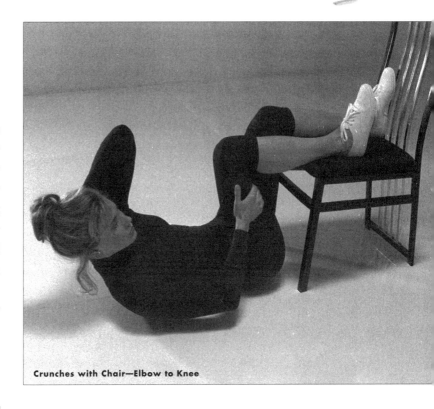

Crunches with Chair—Elbow to Knee

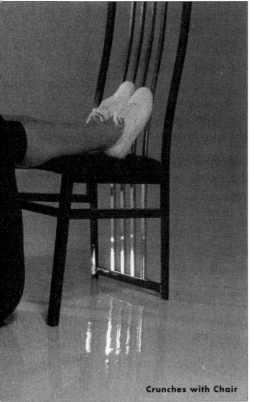

Crunches with Chair

Switch sides. This time bring your left knee forward and lift your right shoulder and elbow up to your left knee.

Do 20 reps with your right elbow to complete 1 set. Release your knees so your feet and calves are once again resting on the chair seat.

Crunches with Hands on Chair

Now lift both hands and place them on the chair between your legs. Look toward your knees and pull in on your abs as you lift your shoulders, sliding your hands forward on

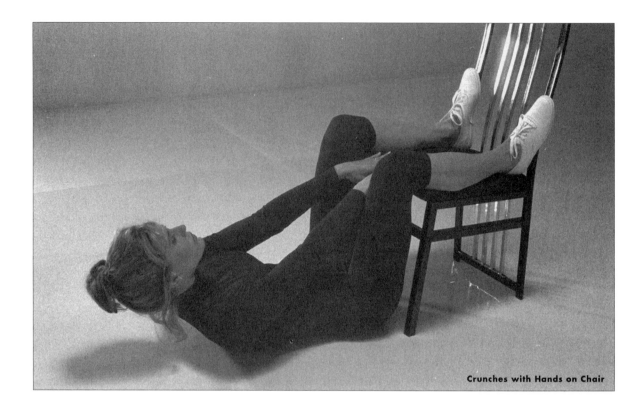

Crunches with Hands on Chair

the chair seat. Lower. Do not take your hands off the chair; keep sliding them forward and back.

Do 20 reps to complete 1 set. Release your hands and bring them back behind your head.

Crunches with Chair—Pelvic Tilt

Now lift your upper body toward your quads. Tilt your pelvis and exhale as you lift in 1 count and then lower.

Do 20 reps to complete 1 set.

Vertical Leg Crunches

Bring your legs up off the chair and extend them straight up with your toes pointed. Now lift your upper body toward your knees and bring in your legs a little so you work the lower abs here, too.

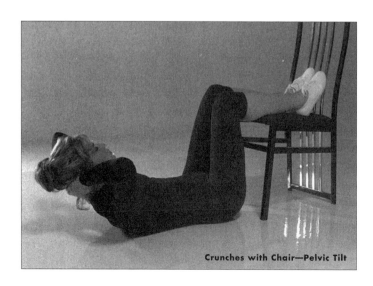

Crunches with Chair—Pelvic Tilt

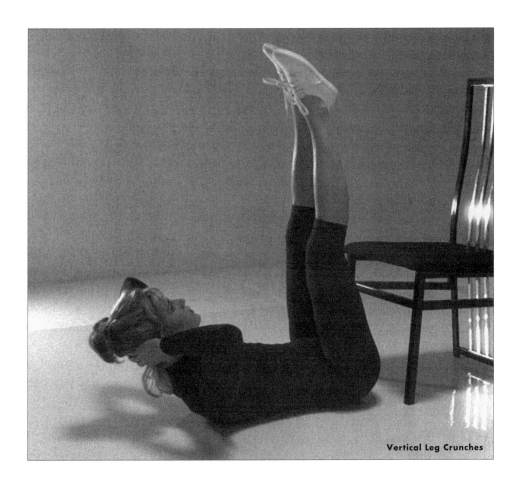

Vertical Leg Crunches

Do 20 reps to complete 1 set and return your feet and calves to the chair.

Crunches with Chair—Pelvic Tilt

Lift your upper body toward your quads. Lift up, tilting your pelvis and exhaling as you lift in 1 count and lower.

Do 10 reps to complete 1 set.

Pulses

Do 10 more pelvic tilts, pulsing 3 times at the top of each crunch.

You did it! Congratulations! The hard part is done.

Cool-Down

Now move on to the cool-down stretches, which are on page 51.

Finish with some applause. You deserve it.

WEEK 6 SUMMARY

Exercise	Reps	Sets
Superset:		
Overhead Press	15	2
Triceps Dips	15	2
Biceps Curls—Angled	15	1
Hammerhead Curls	15	1
Superset:		
Rear Deltoids	15	2
Front Raise	15	2
Triceps Extension—Palm Up	15 right/15 left	2
Superset:		
Three-Count Pliés	8	1
Plié with Pulses	8	1
Pliés	8	1
Plié with Pulses	8	1
Two-Count Lunges	8 right/8 left/8 alternating	1
Hamstrings	10 right/10 left	1
Hamstrings with Pulses	10 right/10 left	1
Three-Count Hamstrings	10 right/10 left	1
Toe Taps	20 right/20 left	2
Left-to-Right (and Right-to-Left) Taps	15 left/15 right	2
Wrap-Leg Calf Raise	15 right/15 left	1
Calf Stretch	hold 8 counts each side	1
Push-Ups—Elbows In	15	3
Toe-to-Side Back Stretch	hold 8 counts each side	

WEEK 6 SUMMARY, CONTINUED

Exercise	Reps	Sets
Superset:		
Side Leg Lift—Knee to Chest	15 right/15 left	1
Vertical Leg Raise	10 left/10 right	1
Vertical Leg Raise with Pulses	10 left/10 right	1
Bottom Leg Lift with Pulses	15 right/15 left	1
Crunches with Chair	20	1
Crunches with Chair—Elbow to Knee	20 left/20 right	1
Crunches with Hands on Chair	20	1
Crunches with Chair—Pelvic Tilt	20	1
Vertical Leg Crunches	20	1
Crunches with Chair—Pelvic Tilt	10	1
Pulses	10	1

10

Applause and the Encore

Your Primetime Body: Keeping the Ratings High

Is the applause still ringing in your ears? It should be. The sixth week of our program is tough but if you toughed it out, we suggest you stick with it as the blueprint for future workouts.

The important thing is to keep doing our exercises. Pick a week's workout that you like and repeat it with weights and more reps. Of course, you can follow the sixth week and repeat it. Mix and match exercises from different weeks to come up with your own workout. Add more weight for your upper body workout. Try using weights on your legs for your lower body workout. Increase reps with heavier weights.

Just make sure you keep appointments with yourself at least four times a week for 35 minutes to an hour—or more!

Aside from exercising, there are other things you can do to keep yourself fit and healthy. Take breathing breaks throughout the day. Exhale so that your abs contract, and inhale pulling in on your abs. Not only will you keep strengthening your abs but you'll feel more relaxed, too.

Of course, you have to watch what you eat. Eat lots of fiber and complex carbohydrates, little fat, and moderate amounts of protein, and drink plenty of water.

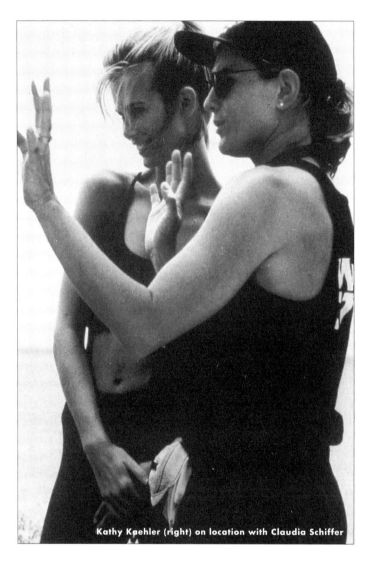

Kathy Kaehler (right) on location with Claudia Schiffer

Don't keep fattening foods in the house. But don't deprive yourself either. If you want a cookie, eat one—not the whole box.

Organize yourself so that when you come home from work there is something healthy already prepared for dinner. That way you won't be reaching for something quick and not so healthy.

You won't be helping yourself if you skip meals. Your body needs fuel just like a car. In order to burn fat, you need to eat.

Walk to the store instead of driving, climb the stairs instead of taking the elevator. Go on an exercise date instead of a movie date. Invite friends over to exercise instead of eating lunch. Ask for exercise equipment as birthday gifts or anniversary gifts.

Find a picture of a model or actress you admire and use that picture as inspiration—your spark to finding your own role as a sleek and healthy primetime body. But remember, you are the outstanding character in your personal show. For you, the best inspiration is to be the best you can be.

If you have temporary setbacks, don't be too hard on yourself. It happens. If you miss your workout appointment, remember how great you feel when you do work out and use that thought as incentive to get back to where you want to be.

Even Michelle Pfeiffer has a pair of test jeans. When they feel a little snug, she counts her calories more closely and she does more lunges! Even the fittest and most beautiful women have to keep working at staying in shape.

We trained Claudia Schiffer, the top supermodel, for her exercise videos. Claudia is a woman who is used to being complimented on her natural beauty. But after she began working out, doing many of the same exercises you've been doing, the people who knew her the best couldn't get over what a difference her workouts had made to her body.

She shaped her entire body, giving great definition to her legs and her upper body. What's even more important, she found new pride in the compliments she received for having achieved her new look through hard work and dedication. Claudia is now taking her weights with her when she's on the road and using them to work her butt, arms, and legs into great shape.

You can do it, too. When you hear those compliments, let them motivate you. When you feel sore from a workout, let it motivate you. When you feel too tired to work out, work out.

It's your primetime body—it's up to you to keep the ratings high. Follow our program and the applause will keep coming.

Good luck!

About the Authors

Cynthia Tivers is a Hollywood writer, director, and producer. She has contributed to many television shows, including "Good Morning America," "Lifestyles of the Rich and Famous," "PM Magazine," and a number of documentaries, specials, and talk shows. In addition to doing celebrity interviews for the Showtime networks, she has written numerous articles for national magazines and is the author of the best-selling book *World Class Legs*.

Kathy Kaehler is one of the hottest personal trainers in Hollywood today. Her celebrity client list includes some of the best-known stars in the world. Michelle Pfeiffer, Meg Ryan, Candice Bergen, Melanie Griffith, Beverly D'Angelo, and Sarah Jessica Parker are only some of the celebrity clients she has trained. Kathy uses her expertise in fitness and weight loss to develop programs for her clients that are effective and easy to follow. Her fitness system is featured on the Kathy Kaehler Fitness System video, and she is featured in the Claudia Schiffer exercise video series.